To Nobbie
    With Love
        From Nobbie,
        For to keep
        Nobbie Cats
            Well + happy.

                (christmas 1978.)

COLLINS A to Z of CAT CARE

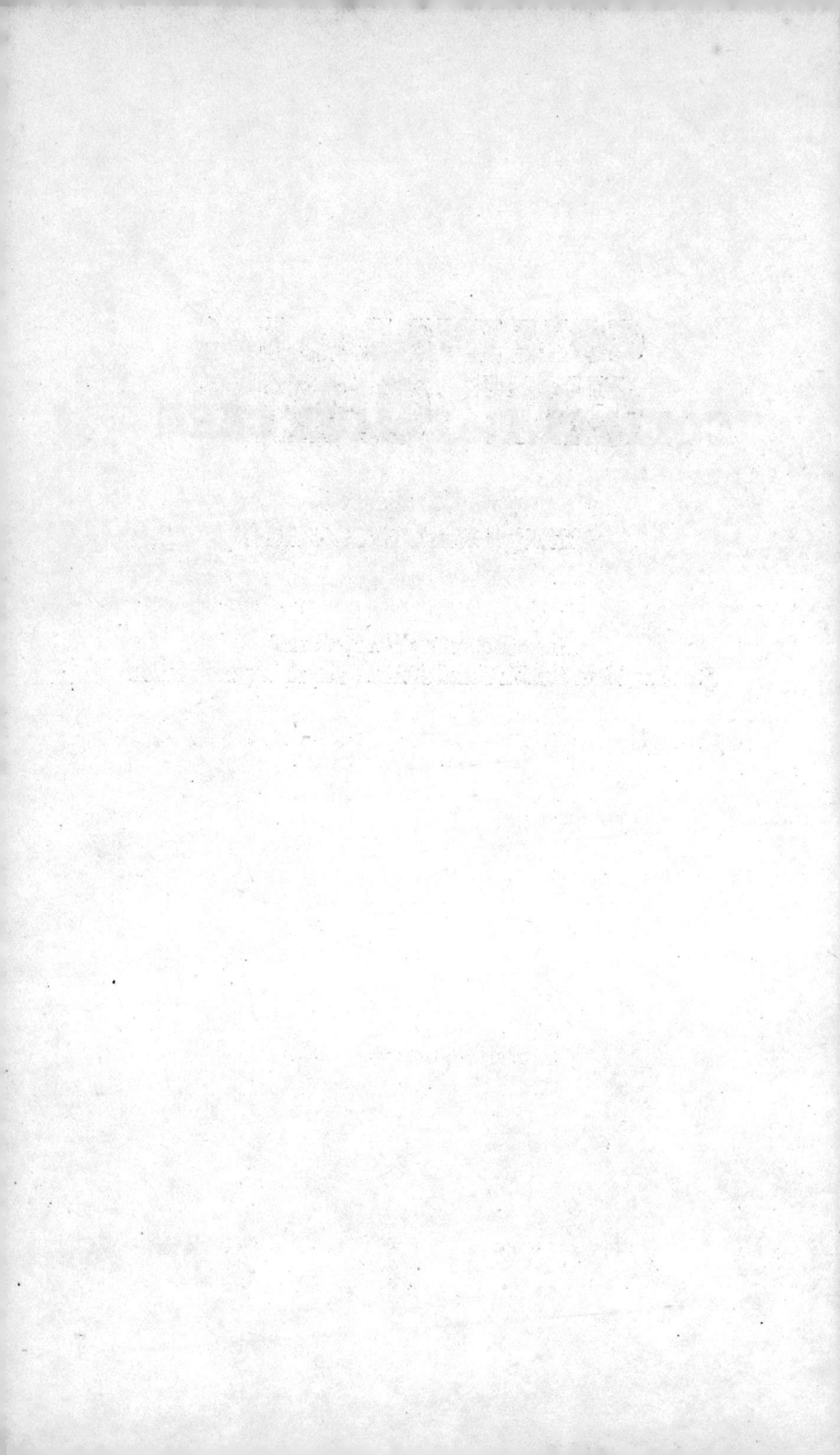

COLLINS A to Z of
CAT CARE

by Stephen Schneck
with Nigel Norris BVSC MRCVS

Introduction by Henry Carter
Past President British Small Animal Veterinary Association

Collins · Glasgow and London

First published 1975
Published by
William Collins Sons and Co. Ltd, Glasgow and London

Copyright © Robert Gurland and Nigel Norris 1975

Illustrations by Kay Marshall

Cover photograph by courtesy of Spectrum

Printed in Great Britain

ISBN 0 00 434577 0

Dedication

To my son Matthew
SS

Acknowledgements

M D Corner B Vet Med MRCVS
Dr P G C Bedford PhD B Vet Med MRCVS
and Caroline

Introduction

One of the many problems facing veterinary surgeons is how to explain, in non-technical language, what is wrong with a pet animal so that the owner can understand and, if possible, help the healing process. The layman can only be expected to have a superficial knowledge of anatomy and physiology, and the rapid advances in diagnosis and treatment in recent years have made the gulf between professional advisor and client even wider.

Veterinarians in small-animal practice soon gain experience in explaining, as simply as possible, what may be a very complex condition. Nevertheless, most of us have felt the need for an up-to-date book compiled especially for the pet owner. *Collins A to Z of Cat Care*, written by a pet owner in collaboration with a practising veterinary surgeon, neatly fills this gap. Factually correct, the information is presented in clear everyday language which will give useful guidance to even the most inexperienced owner with little or no knowledge of biology.

In many parts of the world, a dog or cat owner may be far from the nearest veterinarian, and though in some countries flying doctor services are available, the 'flying vet' is, as yet, a luxury pet owners cannot afford. In these remote areas antibiotics and other medicines are available, but they are of little use without some knowledge and advice on how to use them. In the United Kingdom, and in many other countries, antibiotics etc are (quite rightly) available only on the prescription of a member of the veterinary profession. There are, however, many simple and effective remedies which can be used before professional advice is sought, or when it is not possible to get immediate treatment from a vet. This book helps the owner to cope with both situations and also gives the basic rules for prompt and effective first-aid in emergencies.

The British Small Animal Veterinary Association, representing veterinary surgeons not only in the UK but all over the world, is most concerned that people should look after their pets in a responsible way. This means caring for the health and welfare of the animal and being alert for any changes which may be signs of impending illness. *Collins A to Z of Cat Care* should be of considerable help in furthering this aim and will, I am sure, be welcomed by both pet owners and veterinary surgeons.

Henry Carter MRCVS
Past President British Small Animal
Veterinary Association

How to use this book

The main entries are arranged alphabetically for quick and easy reference, and within each entry the information is given in a logical sequence of causes, symptoms or description, and treatment, where applicable, to make the process of diagnosing and treating any condition as simple and speedy as possible. For example, if your cat is suffering from bad breath, just look up the entry on 'Bad Breath', and follow the instructions for treatment.

If the condition is a more complex one, and you are not exactly sure what it is, you may wish to consult the index at the beginning of the book. Information is indexed in three ways: under the disease name, under the part of the body affected, and under major symptoms displayed. For instance, conjunctivitis is indexed under 'C', as would be expected, but also under 'Eye' and 'Discharge from the eye' and 'Reddening of the eye'. So if you observe that your cat is suffering from red, discharging eyes, you can easily look up either 'Eye' or 'Discharge from the eye' or 'Reddening of the eye' to find out a possible cause. Check to see if the related conditions described in the entry are present in your cat, thus confirming the condition.

Index

A

Abdomen: 1, 5, 11, 19, 22, 23, 24, 42, 50, 54, 57, 59, 71, 75, 78, 82, 83, 86, 88, 90, 99, 107, 109, 110, 111, 125, 127, 133, 142, 147, 149, 152
abdominal wall, tearing of, 88
abnormal motions, 1, 22
acute, 149
appetite, 11, 54, 86, 109, 110, 125
bloat, 24
blood in the motion, 1, 22
blood in vomit, 23
constipation, 42, 78
diarrhoea, 1, 5, 50, 71, 75, 78, 90, 111
distension of the, 24, 147
flatulence, 24
fluid in the, 133, 152
gastritis, 59
gastroenteritis, 71
hernia, 82
hiccups, 83
indigestion, 149
injuries to the, 88
internal parasites, 153
intestines protruding from the, 88
loss of appetite, 11, 71
loss of weight, 152
lump in the groin, 82
pain in the, 19, 71, 82, 111, 107, 147
rigidity of the, 127
strangulation of the bowel, 24
swelling of the, 133
tenseness of the, 127
tumours of the, 11, 42, 152

vomiting, 57, 59, 71, 78, 99, 111, 142, 149, 152
vomiting of blood, 23
Abdominal enlargement, 117, 133
Abdominal pain, severe: 19, 71, 107, 111, 147
front legs extended, 71
rear legs up, 71
restlessness, 107
seeking out cold places to lie on, 107
Abdominal tumours, 11, 42, 133, 152
Ability to detect vibrations, 46; and see Deafness
Abnormal behaviour, 111
Abnormal bowel movement, 1, 42, 50
blood in faeces, 1
colour, 1
constipation, 1, 42
diarrhoea, 1, 50
hard stool, 1
quantity, 1
soft stool, 1
unusual objects in faeces, 1
worms, 1
Abnormal vaginal discharge, 112
Abortion or Miscarriage, 2, 77
Abrasions, 29, 54
Abscesses: 3, 17, 21, 42
of the ano-rectal passage, 42
of the skin, 17
of the tooth roots, 3
pointing of, 3
specific, 3
swelling of, 3
Absence of tear ducts, 130
Accidental overdose of insulin, see Poisoning
Accidents: 7, 20, 22, 23, 25, 26, 32, 46, 60, 63, 68, 88, 89, 124, 146
car, 7, 25, 32, 146

general, 20, 22, 23, 26, 46, 60, 68, 124
road, 60, 88, 89
with fish hooks, 63
Acetone-smelling breath, see Diabetes
Acid poisoning, 111
Acquired deafness, see Deafness
Acute abdomen, 149
Acute eczema: 54
acute, moist, 54
Acute kidney failure, 111
Acute otitis: 4, 67 (see also Ear mites; Middle ear infection)
acute itching, 4
acute soreness, 4
Agalactia (inability to give milk), 85, 106
at birth of first litter, 85
restless behaviour of kittens, 85
Air sickness, see Motion sickness
Alkali burns, 111
Alkali poisoning, 111
Allergic asthma, 5
chestiness, 5
short-windedness, 5
wheeziness, 5
Allergic dermatitis: 5
red patches, itching, 5
red patches, sore, 5
red patches, weeping, 5
Allergies: 5
allergic asthma, 5
allergic dermatitis, 5
diarrhoea, 5
dribbling, 5
general, 5
hay fever, 5
hives, 5
of the respiratory tract, 5
of the skin, 5, 178
running eyes, 5
skin conditions, 5
swelling of the face, 5
vomiting, 5

T

A to Z Entries

1   Abnormal Bowel Movement

See also **Blood in Bowel Movement**

An abnormal bowel movement is distinguished from a normal one by:

Texture
Hard (constipation).
Soft (diarrhoea).

Colour
Blood in faeces: see a vet – there could be ulcers or tumours.
Too pale: suspect problems with gall bladder or pancreas.
Too dark: could be blood in the bowel movement.

Quantity
More than usual.
Less than usual.

Unusual objects in the movement
i.e. worms, bits of bone.

Odour
Certain intestinal infections may cause a particularly strong odour.

2   Abortion or Miscarriage

Miscarriages are infrequent among cats, but they do occur as the result of an infection, a hormonal imbalance, or an accident, or they are due to poor feeding.

Miscarriage, or abortion, occurs when the foetus is expelled from the uterus before the end of the normal gestation period, which is sixty-three days.

Early symptoms
As the birth process begins, the pregnant cat will show signs of discomfort and restlessness, which will be accompanied by some bleeding from the vulva. This bleeding is followed by a clear discharge from the vulva. Then the miscarriage takes place, usually quite rapidly and painlessly, since the embryos are small and soft.

EMERGENCY
In some instances, fortunately rare, severe haemorrhage occurs during the birth or immediately afterwards. *This is an emergency.*
(i)   Try to staunch the bleeding by applying an absorbent pad to the vagina.
(ii)   Keep the cat calm and quiet.
(iii)   Get professional help without delay.

---

3   Abscesses

Description
An abscess is a collection of pus. There is usually some swelling, accompanied by localized pain and heat. Normally, the swelling grows larger and larger until 'pointing' occurs. When this happens, the abscess softens and finally bursts.

WARNING
Do not squeeze an abscess. Allow it to burst naturally. An abscess is formed by the body in order to wall off an infection. When you squeeze the abscess, you are breaking down the wall and forcing the infection back into the body.

Treatment
Encourage the abscess to point by:
(i)   Bathing it in a hot saline solution.
See **Saline Solution**
(ii)   Applying hot compresses directly over it, for ten minutes at a time, four times a day, until it bursts.
(iii)   When it does burst, wash away the pus with a solution of 2 teaspoons (10 ml) hydrogen peroxide, Dettol, Savlon or TCP added to a pint (500 ml) warm water.
(iv)   With abscesses which do not drain completely, continue bathing every two hours with a saline solution. This keeps the abscess open and draining.
(v)   If the compresses are not effective after forty-eight hours, it may be necessary to lance the abscess. If a vet is not available, the owner may lance the abscess himself. (See below.)

The pus which drains from the abscess is usually a creamy colour, but occasionally the pus is pinkish, and large amounts may be confused with a haemorrhage.

Cats which fight often get abscesses, which usually appear on their faces, at the root of their tails or on their feet.

With cats, 'pointing' does not always take place. Instead of the abscess draining, the infection spreads under the skin, causing large fluctuating swellings or very swollen legs and feet. If this condition (called cellulitis) occurs, professional treatment is necessary.

Technique for lancing
(i)   Boil a single-edged razor for twenty minutes.
(ii)   Clean the skin around the affected area with a disinfecting solution of Cetavlon and surgical spirit: 1 teaspoon (5 ml) of each to 1 pint (500 ml) water.
(iii)   Have an assistant, wearing heavy gloves, hold the cat's head tightly. See **Restraint.**
(iv)   Make a half-inch (1 cm) incision over the softest, reddest part of the swelling.
(v)   Allow the abscess to drain.
(vi)   Dress the wound.

Specific abscesses
The specific abscess is found on the upper tooth roots.

Symptoms
If an abscess keeps recurring below the cat's eye, or along the line of the jaw, examine the cat's mouth. A decayed tooth may be causing the abscess. The abscess itself is a discharging sore which appears on the cat's face.

Treatment
There is no first aid for this condition. Tooth root abscesses require extraction of the tooth and antibiotic treatment. See a vet.

---

4   Acute Otitis

Symptoms
The symptoms may be similar to those of ear mites, but this condition is caused by bacteria rather than parasites, and there will be a good deal of inflammation and soreness.

Treatment
To relieve the acute itching and soreness, pour warm olive oil into the ear. To relieve discomfort, administer an analgesic: give half of a 500 mg Paracetamol tablet per 10 lb (5 kg) body

weight, once only. See **Tablets and Pills: Techniques of Administration.**

These are only temporary measures to be used until professional help is available. Acute otitis cannot be cured at home.

WARNING
If left untreated, this can develop into a middle ear infection.

---

5   Allergies

General
Definition
An allergy is a reaction by the body to a substance to which, by previous exposure, it has become oversensitive.

Causes
These substances include hair from other animals, pollen, drugs, foods, certain detergents and fleas. Individual animals vary in their sensitivity to these causes.

Reaction
The physical reaction may take the form of vomiting, diarrhoea, running eyes, red and itching skin, swollen lips and swollen eyelids. While these symptoms are present in other disease states, they will be accompanied by other symptoms. When they appear on their own, for no obvious reason, suspect an allergy.

Treatment
The best way of treating an allergy, of course, is to remove the cause. In situations where this is not possible, either because the allergen cannot be identified, or because it is in the air – e.g. pollen – then it may be necessary for a vet to treat the allergic cat. While a vet will probably administer antihistamines and corticosteroids, the pet owner should be aware that this is professional treatment and that the indiscriminate use of these or any drugs is very dangerous. Further, the use of human medication in the treatment of animals is doubly dangerous, since strength and dosage varies greatly.

Respiratory Tract: Allergic Asthma
This is not a common condition, but when it does occur it must be treated.

Symptoms
Usually occurs during the summer months. Affected cats become very short winded and chesty.

Treatment
A vet would probably administer antihistamines and adrenaline. This is professional treatment and requires veterinary services.

Respiratory Tract: Hay Fever
Hay fever, an allergy of the upper respiratory tract, nose and throat, is fairly common in cats.

Symptoms
Sneezing, accompanied by running eyes and nose, during periods of high pollen count. (Dates vary with locale.)

Treatment
Antihistamines should be administered by a vet.

Skin: Allergic Dermatitis
Causes
This condition is caused by an allergy to certain foods, synthetic carpet fibres, flea saliva, detergents, etc. Causes vary from cat to cat.

Symptoms
The cat develops sore, weeping, itching red patches, which often appear along the spine.
   If left untreated, the condition will not improve.

Treatment
The object of the treatment is to break the itch scratch cycle.
(i)   Shampoo the cat once a week with a selenium based shampoo such as Selsun.
(ii)   Liberal amounts of soothing lotion, such as calamine lotion, should be applied to the affected area twice a day.
(iii)   If the allergic dermatitis is caused by fleas, then as well as treating the dermatitis, get rid of the fleas.
(iv)   Prevent scratching, if necessary, by bandaging the feet.

Skin: Nettlerash
Causes
Poison ivy; stinging nettles; insect bites or stings.

Symptoms
This allergic reaction is quite rare in cats. The effect is very sudden. The eyelids and face become swollen and puffy, clearly defined raised patches appear on the cat's body.

Treatment
(i)   If the cat is not in great discomfort, treatment may not be necessary. Most cases clear up in six to eight hours.
(ii)   If the condition persists after twenty-four hours, seek professional advice.

---

6   Amputation

Amputation is the removal of one or more limbs, either surgically or traumatically.

Surgical amputation
Severe fractures, bone cancers, or very severe cases of arthritis sometimes make amputation necessary.

Many cat owners are naturally reluctant to allow this operation, even when the cat's life is at stake. Some owners would apparently rather have their pets put down than have them hobbling about on three legs. If this reluctance is analysed, it usually turns out that the main objection is to 'the way it will look'. Owners faced with this decision should know that cats learn quite rapidly to compensate for a missing limb, and are able to manage very well on three legs.

Traumatic amputation
This occurs during accidents. A tourniquet must be applied immediately (see **Tourniquets**). Then wrap the cat in a towel or coat to keep it warm and minimize the effects of shock while the cat is being transported to the vet.

If possible, have someone telephone the vet so that he can have the necessary transfusions ready when the cat arrives. See **Car Accidents: Moving an Injured Cat.**

---

7   Anaemia

This is a blood condition characterized by the reduction of the oxygen-carrying capacity of the blood. There are three main causes of anaemia:

1 Loss of blood.
2 Blood destruction (due to infections such as feline infectious anaemia: microscopic blood parasites).
3 Poor blood formation (iron deficiency).

Symptoms
The cat is lethargic; it shows no enthusiasm. Its pulse is rapid. The animal is unnaturally pale around its eyes and nose and gums. See **Pulse Taking**.

Of course, to an extent, the symptoms vary from one situation to another. A cat suffering from a debilitating disease will develop this pallor gradually, while a cat suffering from a haemorrhaging gastric ulcer or one involved in a car accident will suddenly become very pale around the mucous membranes.

A cat suffering from feline infectious anaemia will have a temperature fluctuating from very high to normal. See **Temperature Taking**.

Treatment
All anaemic animals need professional treatment, since anaemia is almost always symptomatic of other diseases or deficiencies. If professional help is not immediately available for chronic anaemia, administer ferrous sulphate tablets (obtainable from chemists) until you can have your pet seen by a vet. Give half a 30 mg tablet once a day.

---

8 Analgesics

Analgesics are pain-killers. When administering them, pay careful attention to dosages. Only administer when the cat is in acute discomfort. You have to know your pet's normal behaviour pattern well in order to gauge accurately the degree of pain.

When to administer
If the cat is in obvious pain or discomfort.

Dosage
Half of a 500 mg Paracetamol tablet per 10 lb (5 kg) body weight, twice a day.

WARNING
Never administer aspirin or codeine preparations.

9   Anthropomorphism

Next to sheer ignorance, anthropomorphism is probably the second-ranking cause of improper home medical treatment.

Anthropomorphism, in this context, is the fallacy of attributing human behaviour and mentality to cats. While it is perfectly normal to speak of an animal as being 'nearly human', actually believing it can lead to serious errors of judgement, which in turn can lead to incorrect medical treatment. If we think of a cat as a human being we cannot properly observe and evaluate the animal's behaviour. In many instances this makes it impossible to reach a correct diagnosis.

Cats have their own psychology, their own pattern of behaviour, and their own set of reactions. If we are to treat cats intelligently, we must begin by thinking of them as cats and not as four-legged people.

10   Antibiotics

Antibiotics, drugs which kill the germs that cause infections, should only be administered by a vet. They are most effective when administered during the early stage of the infection. (Antibiotics are not usually effective against virus infections.)

Ideally, if your cat has an infectious disease, the particular strain of bacteria that is causing it should be identified and the specific antibiotic administered.

Unfortunately, disease states are rarely ideal, so a broad-spectrum antibiotic is administered.

If there is no response within twenty-four hours, another broad-spectrum antibiotic is used, and possibly another, until a satisfactory response occurs.

11   Appetite

Increase of appetite
A noticeable increase of appetite suggests:
1   Abdominal tumours.
2   Diseases which prevent the food from being absorbed.
3   Neutered cats tend to deposit more fat.
4   Simple greed, which may be due to a neurotic condition or, in certain extreme cases, brain damage.
5   Pregnancy.

Treatment
Depends upon the cause. In the case of desexed cats, simply
feed them less. The first, second and fourth causes are beyond
the scope of home treatment, and should be treated profession-
ally. The fifth cause treats itself.

Loss of appetite
It is not unusual for a cat to go off its food for twenty-four
hours. But if the cat refuses food after twenty-four hours, loss
of appetite may be a symptom of something else. Check for:
1 Generalized disease: the cat is apathetic, listless. Its coat is
dull. It may be feverish. The cat acts and looks ill. These are
very broad and general symptoms, and are one more good
reason why owners should observe their cats while in good
health. Deviations from the norm are easy to recognize for
those familiar with their cat's normal behaviour and appearance.
2 Tartar on the teeth can cause the cat pain when chewing.
3 Foreign body in the mouth, such as splinter of bone between the teeth.
4 Sore mouth or sore throat.

Treatment
The procedure for examining the mouth is to get the cat into
a good light or use a flashlight to examine the mouth and
throat for sores, tartar, inflammation or obstructions. If none
of these are observed, then take the cat's temperature. If it is
above normal, consult a vet. See **Temperature Taking.**
(i) Loss of appetite due to a generalized disease must be
treated by a vet.
(ii) If the cat's teeth reveal an accumulation of tartar, see
Tartar on the Teeth for treatment.
(iii) If a foreign body is blocking the mouth or throat, open
the cat's mouth and remove the object. See **Opening a Cat's
Mouth.**
(iv) To check for a sore throat, gently feel around the cat's
larynx. If the throat is sore, the cat will cough. In this case, a
vet should be consulted.
(v) If there does not seem to be anything wrong with the cat,
but it still refuses to eat, try to tempt it with a change of diet.
Try succulent treats like boiled, boned chicken, strong
cheeses, kippers, or essence of beef (Brands Essence).
    Cats will refuse to eat food that they cannot smell, so when a
cat will not eat, check for cat flu symptoms. See **Cat Flu.**

12   Artificial Respiration

Artificial respiration does the work of normal breathing: shifting the air in and out of the animal's lungs. Artificial respiration should be administered as soon as it is observed that the cat is not breathing. Within two to three minutes after breathing stops, the cat will be beyond recovery.

Technique (see illustration)
(i)   Lay the cat on its right side.
(ii)   Open the cat's mouth and check to be sure that there are no obstructions to breathing. If there are obstructions, pull then out with your finger. Also be sure that the tongue is clear of the back of the throat.
(iii)   Place the flat of both hands below the shoulder blade and over the ribs.
(iv)   Press down firmly to empty the lungs.
(v)   Release. The lungs should fill as the chest wall returns to its normal position.
(vi)   Repeat the pressing down and releasing the pressure every five seconds until the cat is breathing on its own again.
(vii)   These movements should be brisk and forceful. Press down hard; release suddenly.

Mouth-to-mouth respiration
It is simple enough. Just hold the cat's mouth closed and blow into its nostrils. Wait and allow the chest to empty. Repeat.

The idea is to inflate the animal's lungs with air, so that they function of their own accord.

If the cat does not respond immediately, remember, as long as you can hear a heartbeat, there is hope!

Swinging technique
(i)   Slap the cat sharply on its side once or twice.
(ii)   Then lift the cat by its hind legs. Extend your arms and swing the animal back and forth ten times (see illustration 2). Wait a few seconds for a gasp. If there is none, then swing the cat again.

When you swing a cat, as described, the weight of the abdominal contents will contract and expand the lungs. If, after four such swinging sessions, the cat is still not breathing, administer mouth-to-mouth respiration.

(i) *and* (ii)

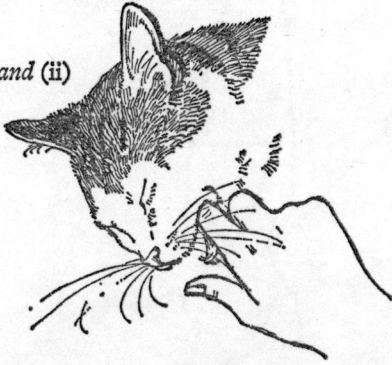

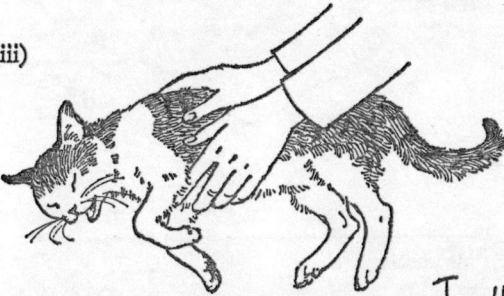

(iv)

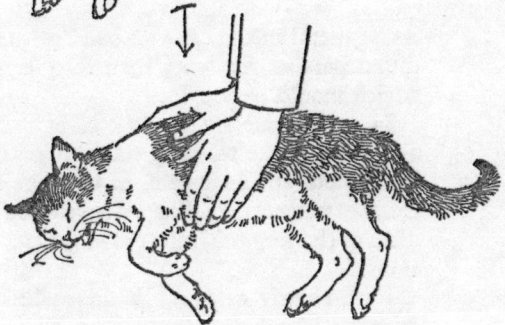

(v)

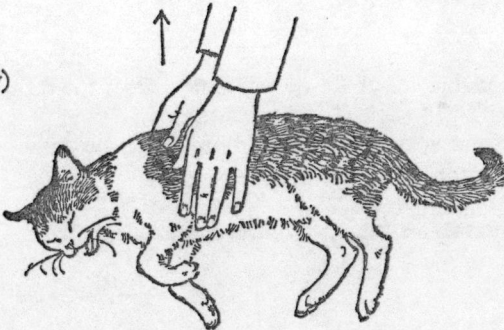

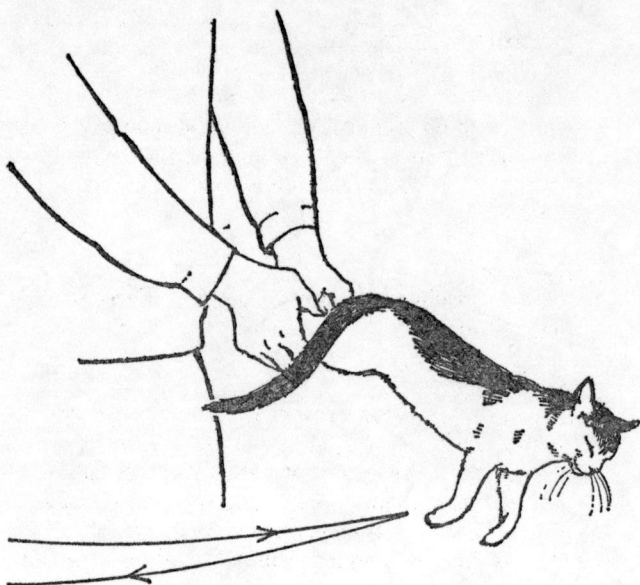

13   Bad Breath (Halitosis)

As a general rule, a cat with bad breath is not well. If the condition persists for more than forty-eight hours, professional advice should be sought.

In cats under six months of age, bad breath sometimes accompanies the teething stage. It may also indicate a worm infestation. In older cats, bad breath suggests a number of disease states: tonsillitis, stomach infection, stomatitis, an ulcer of the stomach, infected or broken teeth, labial eczema or sinusitis.

With elderly cats, continuing halitosis usually indicates a degree of chronic kidney failure.

Treatment
First, as far as possible, check for disease states. Does the cat act as if it is sick? Is it feverish? Is it apathetic?

Once these disease states have been eliminated as possible causes for bad breath, treat the condition by administering chlorophyll tablets or charcoal tablets. Give one tablet a day. Continue the treatment even after the bad breath has been cleansed.

14   Baldness (Alopecia)

Causes
This condition is not uncommon in cats and may occur without any visible cause. Baldness may be the result of an iodine deficiency, a hormonal imbalance or certain generalized illnesses.

Symptoms
The hair begins to fall out in patches. These patches may or may not itch.

Treatment
(i)   Apply a solution made by mixing 1 teaspoon of iodine crystals with 1 pint (500 ml) glycerine. Shake well until the crystals have dissolved. Saturate a piece of cotton wool with the solution and apply directly to the bald patches.
(ii)   Continue treatment for five to six weeks.
(iii)   If there is no improvement, obtain professional help.

15   Bandaging

Bandages are used to:
1   Stop bleeding.
2   Support injured legs.
3   Prevent the cat from biting at its injuries.
4   Reduce swelling.
5   Prevent bacteria from entering the wound and causing infection.

Preferred type of bandage
The easiest type of bandage to use is the roller bandage, available in 12 ft (3.5 m) and 15 ft (4.5 m) lengths and a variety of widths.

For bandaging cats, the most useful width is the 2 in (5 cm) or 3 in (7.5 cm) roller bandage. For wounds on the trunk of the cat, the 4 in (10 cm) bandage is suggested.

Bandaging the eye (see illustration 3)
Technique
(i)   Place a moist gauze pad over the affected eye.
(ii)   Wind the bandage around the animal's head, leaving the ears in their normal position.

(i)

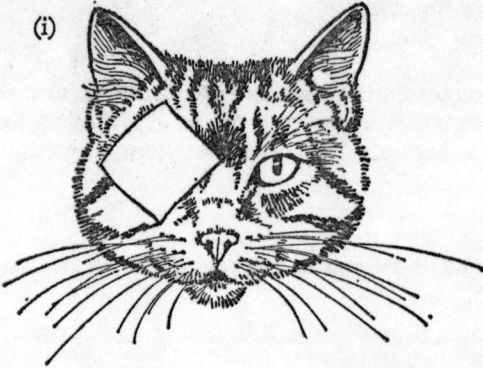

(ii)

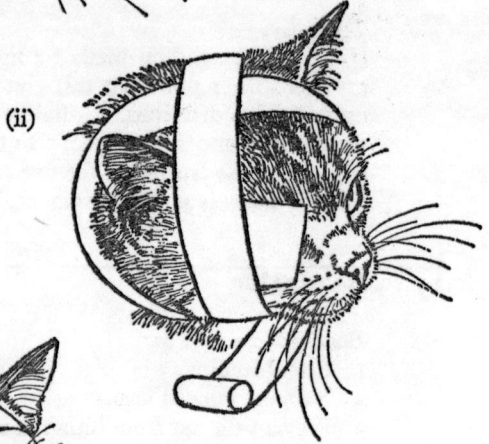

(iii)

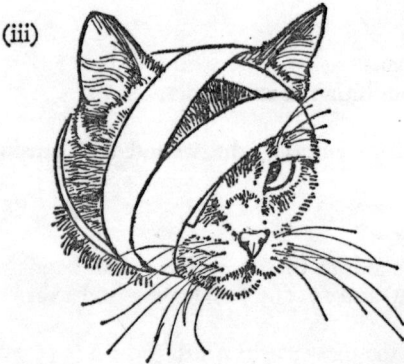

(iv)

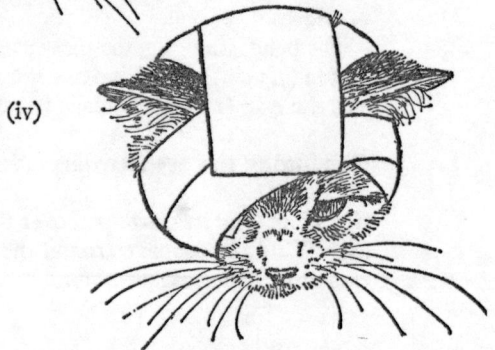

(i)

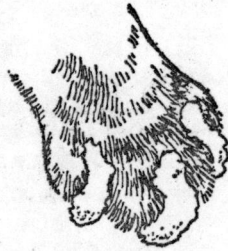

(ii)

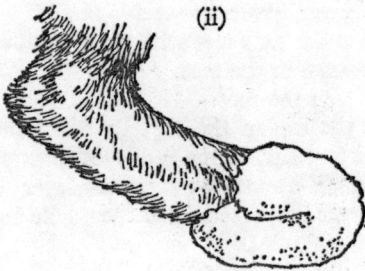

(iii)

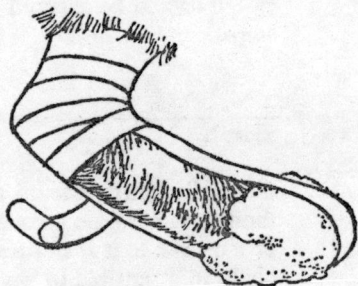

(iv)

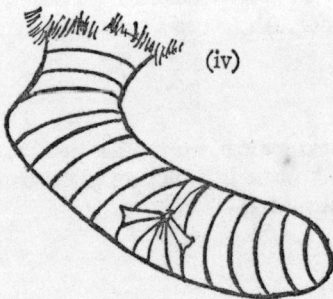

(iii)   Extend the bandage forward to cover the gauze dressing over the affected eye.

(iv)   Anchor the bandage with a strip of 2 in (5 cm) or 3 in (7.5 cm) elastoplast, placed at the top of the cat's head.

(v)   Take care not to wind the bandage too tightly, and be sure that it does not interfere with the cat's breathing.

Bandaging the leg (see illustration 4)
Technique
When bandaging the leg, you should bandage the foot as well, in order to prevent swelling and tissue damage.

(i)   Pack the spaces between the cat's toes with small wads of cotton wool, to prevent damage to the toes.

(ii)   Wrap cotton wool around the foot.

(iii)   Begin bandaging at the top of the leg; go down the front of the leg, around the foot and up the back (see illustration). Then wind the bandage around the leg, each layer of bandage overlapping the preceding layer, until the whole leg is covered.

(iv)   Tie off the bandage.

(v)   The bandage should be wound firmly enough not to slip, but not so tightly that it stops the circulation, unless it is a pressure bandage intended to stop a haemorrhage, in which case it should be checked every 30 minutes until the bleeding stops.

---

16   Birth

Generally, birth occurs sixty-three days after conception, though on occasion a queen may give birth up to a week early or late. While it is not necessary to have a vet present at the birth, it is sensible to have a pregnant cat examined by a vet prior to the event. Fortunately, cats are quite expert at home deliveries, but it is a good idea to observe the birth, if possible, just in case something goes wrong. Also, keep a vet's telephone number handy.

Signs of appraoching birth
1   Approximately six hours before birth, the mother becomes restless and begins preparing a place in which to give birth (usually the most inconvenient place!)
2   Vomiting may occur.

3 The cat's body temperature drops three degrees to about 98°F (36°C).
4 The vulva becomes enlarged and pinkish.
5 The pelvic ligaments slacken, causing some loss of co-ordination of the hind legs.

Labour

1 Within an hour before birth, the mother grows increasingly nervous, and may start glancing at her flanks. There are occasional contractions of the abdomen, becoming more frequent.
2 The mother lies down as the contractions become more frequent. As the foetus enters the pelvis, there is definite straining. The water bag, which looks like a black grape, appears at the vulva.
3 The mother will lick the water bag to rupture it. After the water breaks, the nose and feet of the kitten will appear, protruding from the vulva.
4 After violent expulsive efforts by the mother, the infant animal is born. Often the mother will cry out as the kitten's head comes through.
5 The final stage is the expulsion of the remaining membranes from the womb. This can occur as long as one hour after the kittens have been born.

Complications

(i) If there is more than a two-minute delay after the head and front legs are out, the kitten should be gently pulled out. Use a towel to grip without slipping. Grip as high as you can. It is essential that the kitten is extracted as quickly and as carefully as possible.
(ii) Some kittens are born head first, some tail first. Both positions are normal, but if the kitten is born tail first, it should come out fairly rapidly. After the water has broken, the kitten should be out in ten minutes. If the kitten is not out in this time, telephone a vet.
(iii) If the kitten is born with the membranes surrounding it still intact, and the mother does not remove them, do this *quickly* yourself.
(iv) Every kitten should be checked immediately to make sure that its mouth is free of mucus, enabling it to breathe freely.
(v) If breathing does not occur at once, rub the kitten briskly with a rough towel. If this does not work, try mouth-to-mouth

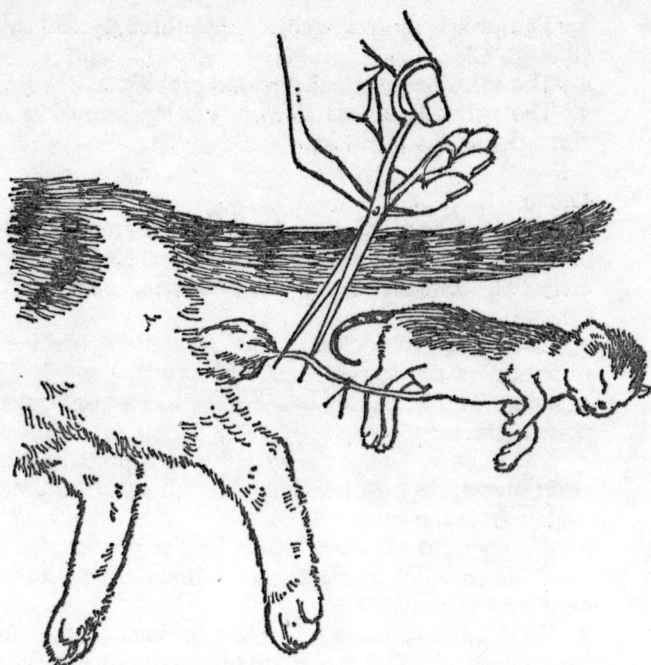

respiration (see **Artificial Respiration**), or place the kitten in a bowl of warm water and then plunge it into a bowl of cold water.

(vi)   Once breathing has begun, put the kitten back with its mother and let her lick it dry.

(vii)   The mother may try to eat the membranes, but allow her to eat only one set, or she may develop diarrhoea. See **Mother Cat eating her Kittens**.

Umbilical Cord
The umbilical cord should break when the kitten comes out of the membranes. If it does not break, tie it off with clean boiled cotton, 2 in (5 cm) from the kitten, and cut it on the side of the knot farthest away from the kitten.

After birth
After the kitten is born, more membranes may be expelled. A green discharge, several hours after birth, is quite normal.

The size of a litter normally varies from one to six kittens. Of course, there are exceptions to every rule, and the current world record, according to the Guinness Book of Records, is thirteen kittens in a single litter.

If a queen seems nervous or overprotective towards her newly-born litter, or if she objects to strangers or even family handling her young, humour her. Keep the strangers and the rest of the family away from the kittens. Of course, children are usually the main offenders, and it is difficult to refuse them the delights of handling newly-born kittens, but if the kittens' mother shows any resentment, this must be done. After all, they are *her* kittens.

---

17   Bites, Fight Wounds

There are two types of wounds received from animal bites: lacerated wounds and puncture wounds.

Lacerated wounds
The wound is jagged. The skin is torn. There may be profuse bleeding.

Treatment
(i)   Clean the wound with Cetavlon or soap and water.
(ii)   Check that the wound has drained and that there is no infection left. If the wound is discharging pus, it is still infected.
(iii)   If the wound is very large, it may require stitches.

Puncture wounds
These are small holes in the skin, but they are quite deep and are often accompanied by bruising. Puncture wounds are the most serious type of bite-wound. If a puncture wound is left untreated, the skin will heal, but an abscess will form underneath.

Treatment
(i)   Clean the area around the wound with soap and water, or Cetavlon and water.
(ii)   Puncture wounds almost always become infected, so get professional advice within twenty-four hours.

18   Bitten Tongue

Symptoms
Profuse bleeding from the mouth.

Treatment
A bitten tongue may sound a rather minor mishap, but if the bleeding is very heavy, then it must be considered an emergency. Since the tongue is constantly moist and moving, it is difficult for a blood clot to form, so bleeding is continuous and, if the cut is deep enough, the cat can bleed to death. Fortunately, it would take at least twenty-four hours for this to happen, which gives plenty of time to get the animal to a vet.

If it is possible, that is, if the cat will allow it, hold the tongue in a cotton wool pad to reduce the bleeding while you are transporting the animal to the vet.

19   Bladder Infection (Cystitis)

A fairly common condition in cats.

Symptoms
1   Blood, or traces of blood, in the urine.
2   Passing small amounts of urine.
3   Abdominal pain.
4   In later stages, the urine will be heavily stained with blood. As the disease progresses, pure blood will be passed.
5   Unfortunately for home diagnosis, cats are so discreet in their urination habits that they may pass traces of blood in their urine without the owner noticing it.
6   The classic symptom of cystitis in a cat is seen when the animal is in its litter box straining to pass urine. The position is exactly the same as when trying to pass a motion, but the constipated cat rarely strains, while the cat with cystitis does.

Treatment
If the bladder infection is suspected, do not feed the cat until professional help is available. In the event that it takes more than twenty-four hours to get to a vet, allow the cat access to all the water it wants to drink. Keep its drinking bowl full.

NOTE
There is some evidence to suggest that the feeding of some dry

cat foods is responsible for urethral obstruction. It is thought that the magnesium salts in these commercial preparations causes sedimentation in the urine and subsequent urethral obstruction.

20 Blindness

Progressive blindness
This condition is fairly common. It is usually the result either of old age or of the formation of cataracts, which could be due to diabetes.

Sudden blindness
A result either of a stroke or an accident in which the brain or the eyes themselves have been injured.

Temporary blindness
This occurs during infections of the clear part of the eye, i.e. keratitis. These infections, if not properly treated, can give rise to milkiness and eventually to ulceration of the cornea (corneal ulcer).

If ulceration occurs, immediate professional treatment is vital. *Do not bathe the eye.* Corneal ulcers take a long time to heal, and the cat may be left with a black scar on the cornea.

Treatment
If you suspect that your cat is going blind (and of course the symptoms are painfully obvious: bumping into things, inability to recognize people at a distance, etc.), the first thing to do is to have your cat examined by a vet. He will be able to give you a definite diagnosis, and, in the case of cataracts, will possibly improve the condition by surgery or enzyme injections.

But even if the condition is irreversible, the cat owner should be aware that blindness need not be the end of the animal's life. When the eyes fail, the other senses develop to compensate. Blind animals, as a rule, have a much better sense of hearing and of smell than do sighted animals. By the time the cat is completely blind, it will know its way around the house. Blind animals, on the whole, manage remarkably well. They just need a little extra care.

21   Blood Blister on the Ear (Haematoma)

Description
A thick, fluctuating, irregular swelling usually found on the inside of the ear flap, but the outside of the ear flap may be involved as well. The blister itself is painless and rather firmer than an abscess.

These blisters come up quite suddenly, usually as the result of a blow or a bite, as the sequel to an ear mite infection, or from an irritation which causes constant scratching. Such an irritation might be caused by an infection in the ear, in which case it will be accompanied by pus coming from the ear canal.

Treatment
If the blister is the result of an ear infection and is small, then leave it alone and treat the infection.

Treatment for a persistent blister
(i)   If the blister has not disappeared after three or four days, minor surgery will be required to drain, curette and suture it.
(ii) If the persistent blister is fairly small (approximately $\frac{1}{2}$ inch (1 cm) in diameter), you can drain it yourself. Sterilize a needle by boiling it for twenty minutes; wash your hands; prick the blister on the inside of the ear flap with the sterile needle and allow it to drain naturally.
(iii) With large blisters, it is advisable to seek professional assistance.

Blood blisters, while not serious in themselves, can easily cause permanent disfigurement of the ear. The best first aid is to keep them bandaged and taped to the animal's head to prevent it from worrying them and making them worse than they already are. If the cat persists in worrying them, use an Elizabethan Collar to discourage this. See **Elizabethan Collar.**

22   Blood in Bowel Movement

A small amount of blood in the faeces is seen from time to time in all meat-eating animals. Larger amounts of blood, however, are not normal and should not be ignored.

Causes
Blood in the faeces may be the result of a rectal impaction,

bones, or it may be caused by tumours of the rectum or accidents.

Symptoms
1   If the blood found in the faeces is bright red and fresh, it comes from the anal region.
2   If the blood is black, it comes from the intestines.
3   Consider the source or location of the bleeding when attempting to diagnose the cause.

Treatment
Unless the cause can be easily identified and treated, such as bones or a simple cut, have your cat examined by a vet.

---

23   Blood in Vomit

Causes
Fresh blood in your cat's vomit may be caused by accidents, tumours, or by foreign bodies which have cut the mouth, throat or gullet.

If the blood found in the vomit is black, then it comes from the stomach or from the small intestine and may be caused by a stomach ulcer or by tumours.

Treatment
There is no home treatment for this condition, since it is not possible for the cat owner to diagnose the cause accurately.

As a temporary measure, the cat should not be fed. A vet should be consulted at once.

---

24   Breaking Wind (Flatulence)

Causes
1   Overweight.
2   Lack of exercise.
3   Dietary imbalance.
4   Bowel infection.

Treatment
(i)   If your cat is elderly, and you have been feeding it one large meal a day, start feeding it two or three smaller meals a day. Be sure you are not overfeeding.

(ii)   Allow the cat more opportunity for exercise.

(iii)   If the cat is always indoors, get toys (mechanical mice, marbles, etc.) and play with your pet.

If reducing the size of meals and increasing the opportunity for exercise does not help, then:

(iv)   Add a teaspoon of charcoal to the cat's food each day.

(v)   Remove liver and heart from the cat's diet.

---

25   Broken Back (Fractured Spine)

Fractures and dislocations of the spinal column almost never occur spontaneously. They are usually the result of some traumatic incident such as a car accident, a fall, or a blow with a stick across the back.

Symptoms

1   The cat will be unable to move its rear limbs.

2   It will be insensitive to pain below the affected portion of the spine.

3   There will be urinary and faecal incontinence and retention.

4   As a general rule, if the animal cannot move both back legs, if there is no response when the toe is firmly pinched and the cat has been involved in an accident, it is a fair assumption that it has a break or fracture of the spine.

5   The cat usually lies with its front legs extended. These same symptoms could also indicate a slipped disc. But the slipped disc occurs spontaneously and not as the result of a traumatic accident.

Treatment

(i)   *If the cat has been hit by a car, do not move it unless it is absolutely necessary.*

(ii)   Telephone a vet, the police or the RSPCA.

(iii)   Wrap the cat in a blanket or coat, and carry it in a basket or box to the vet.

Prognosis

The outlook for cats which suffer fractures and dislocations of the spine is not very hopeful. In the majority of cases, the cat will have to be put down.

Fractures of the tail occur after accidents and in cats confined to small areas.

Fractures at the root of the tail
If the break has taken place at the root of the tail, the whole length of the tail will hang straight down. Also, there will be some pain and swelling at the site of the fracture.

Treatment
The owner should not attempt to treat root fractures. Professional assistance is necessary. If the cat is in pain, administer half a Paracetamol tablet. See **Tablets and Pills: Techniques of Administration.** Then get the cat to a vet.

Fractures along the length of the tail
Fractures of this type are easily identifiable. The tail, up to the site of the fracture, can be moved by the cat, while that portion of the tail beyond the fracture will hang limply.

Treatment
If there should be a delay of more than twenty-four hours before the cat can be seen by a vet, an elastoplast dressing should be applied to support the length of the damaged tail. Tape the break, tight enough to provide support, but not so tight that the circulation is cut off.

Fractures of the tip of the tail
Again, an elastoplast dressing should be taped around the fracture; again, be careful not to tape it too tightly.
It usually takes about two weeks for a tail fracture to mend.

It is important that cats with fractures or suspected fractures of the tail should be examined by a vet. Quite often nerve damage is caused, and that portion of the tail beyond the fracture may have to be removed surgically.

27   **Broken Tooth**

Occasionally a cat breaks its tooth by biting too hard on something harder than its tooth.
This is not an emergency. Of course, the broken tooth may

have to be extracted eventually. But meanwhile there is one consolation: a broken tooth does not hurt. However, very cold or very hard substances can damage the exposed portion of the tooth.

Symptoms
Dribbling. Slight bleeding from the mouth.

---

28   Bronchitis, Excessive Coughing

Symptoms
Excessive coughing, often with phlegm. Sometimes accompanied by a high fever.

Treatment
(i)   First, get a good light and examine the cat's throat to make sure that the cough is not caused by a foreign body in the mouth or throat. See **Foreign Bodies.**
(ii)   Then treat the symptoms as they arise. Treat the cough with a mixture of 1 teaspoon (5 ml) glycerine mixed with 1 teaspoon (5 ml) honey, three times a day. You will probably have to pour this mixture down the cat's throat, so prepare yourself by reading the entry **Force-Feeding.**
(iii)   Give no food for twenty-four hours, then a light diet of fish, rabbit or chicken. If, after forty-eight hours, your cat is still coughing excessively, find a vet.
Bronchitis is common during lung-worm infestations. Obviously, if you think your cat has bronchitis, you should contact a vet. Only in extraordinary circumstances, when a vet is not available, should home treatment be attempted.
(iv)   If there is no fever, administer Diphenhydramine cough medicine: 1 teaspoon (5 ml) twice a day for three days.

---

29   Bruises and Contusions

Description
Bruises and contusions are easy to see on the hairless parts of the animal, where the bruise appears bluish red and is painful to the touch.
If the bruise is under the fur, you will not be able to see it, but you will be able to feel it and to judge by your cat's reaction just how severe it is.

Treatment

(i) Examine the area around the bruise for breaks in the skin; these cuts and abrasions are often seen in association with bruises. If you find any cuts, clean and dress them. See Dressing wounds (Index).

(ii) Apply hot compresses over the bruise for five minutes every two hours. It is helpful to have an assistant hold the cat while you are applying the compresses. See **Restraint.**

(iii) If the cat is suffering marked discomfort, administer half a Paracetamol tablet, once only. See **Tablets and Pills: Techniques of Administration.**

---

30   Burns and Scalds

Burns and scalds are the most common of household accidents, and the cat owner should familiarize himself with the treatment of these mishaps *before* they occur.

A burn is caused by dry heat, such as a flame. A scald is caused by moist heat, such as steam. But the difference is academic, since the symptoms and the treatment are the same.

Treatment

(i) When handling or treating a cat which has been burned, be careful. Burns are very painful, and animals in pain resent being handled. An assistant is essential. See **Restraint.**

(ii) In serious cases, where the cat has been badly burned, treat first for shock by wrapping the cat in a blanket or towel to keep it warm. Then force-feed a solution made by adding 3 teaspoons glucose powder to $\frac{1}{2}$ pint (250 ml) water. See **Force-Feeding.**

(iii) Relieve the pain by administering analgesics (see **Analgesics**).

(iv) Clean the area around the burn with a dilute solution of Cetavlon – 1 teaspoon (5 ml) to 1 pint (500 ml) water – to remove any damaged tissue (burnt or charred skin).

(v) Apply tannic acid jelly (available from chemists) or a solution of strong tea to the burned area. Be sure to let the tea cool before applying it.

(vi) Bandage the area to prevent further loss of fluid. It is this loss of fluid that creates serious problems in burn cases.

(vii) In very severe cases, wrap the animal in a blanket and get it to a vet.

Long-haired cats

If a long-haired cat is burned or scalded, it usually takes two or three days before any signs appear. After this time a sticky green crust forms on the skin. *Do not pull this crust off*. It will come away of its own accord, leaving a large, pinkish, weeping area. If it does not come away, bathe or soak it off. Then the area should be cleaned and dressed. Use a little cod liver oil on a cotton wool pad for the dressing.

Very severe cases

In very severe cases with associated shock, a vet will give stimulants and plasma to combat the loss of fluid. See **Shock; Car Accidents: Moving an Injured Cat.**

Chemical Burns

Causes

Caustic soda; sulphuric acid; hydrochloric acid (spirits of salt); diesel oil, etc. (A note on diesel oil: animals may come into contact with diesel oil if they go under a parked lorry.)

Description

1 A chemical burn resembles a scald. The wound is moist and oozing.
2 The hair around the burn usually sloughs off.
3 If the cat has tried to drink the chemical, there will be sores on its muzzle and tongue.

Treatment

(i) Use soap and water to wash the chemical off the cat's fur and skin.
(ii) For acid burns, apply dilute bicarbonate of soda to the burned area. If the burn was caused by an alkali, such as caustic soda, apply vinegar to the burned area. If you have no idea which chemical caused the burn, play it safe and clean the area with soap and water.
(iii) Apply hydrogen peroxide (available from chemists) directly on to the burn to disinfect it.

---

31   Calcium

The main function of calcium in the diet is to aid the growth and formation of teeth and bones.

Proper amounts of calcium in the diet of kittens is essential.

A lack of calcium will cause rickets, resulting in swollen tender joints, arched back and stiff legs.

Acute calcium deficiency in the lactating cat will produce a condition called **Milk Fever.**

Milk is a natural source of calcium. But a cat suffering from a calcium deficiency needs a concentrated dose and should be fed a solution which is made by adding 1 teaspoon calcium borogluconate powder (available from chemists) to 10 teaspoons (50 ml) water. Shake well until the powder is dissolved. The cat will probably refuse to drink this voluntarily, so the owner should be prepared to force-feed. See **Force-Feeding.**

---

32   Car Accidents: Moving an Injured Cat

First considerations
Do not move the animal any more than you have to. Decide *where* you are going to move the cat to *before* you move it.

Before you move an injured cat
(i)   If the cat is bleeding profusely, try to stop the bleeding before you move the animal. (See below.)
(ii)   Check for a possible fractured spine by pinching the injured cat's toes. If the cat does not register pain, there is a possiblity that the spine is fractured. In this event, do not move the cat unless it is absolutely essential.

Bleeding
If you can, determine whether the bleeding is from an artery or from a vein. This is done by observing the way the blood flows.

Arterial bleeding
If the blood comes out in a pumping fashion, in time with the heartbeat, and is bright red, then it is from an artery and the bleeding must be stopped or the cat will die.

If there is arterial bleeding from a limb, make a tourniquet by wrapping a bandage, handkerchief or necktie around the limb, *above* the injury, and inserting a pencil or a screwdriver into the bandage. Then twist the tourniquet until the bleeding stops. See illustration 14.

Venous bleeding
Blood flowing from a vein flows regularly, as opposed to being

pumped. Also, it is dark red in colour. If the blood is coming from a vein, apply the tourniquet *below* the wound. See illustration 14.

It is important to remember that a tourniquet should not be too tight; just tight enough to stop the bleeding. Loosen the tourniquet every ten minutes to allow the blood to get to the rest of the body.

Bleeding: Emergencies

Unfortunately, there is usually such a mess that you cannot determine whether the blood is flowing or pumping. Often the wounds are on the body, where a tourniquet cannot be applied. So, unless the source of bleeding is obvious and easily tied off, the best thing you can do is the fastest thing. Grab anything – bandages, a torn shirt, a handkerchief, even a packet of tissues – and put it over the wound, holding it there with as much pressure as you can.

Internal bleeding

If the bleeding is internal, or the blood is flowing from the cat's nose or anus, there is nothing you can do except keep the animal still and get it to a vet as fast as possible. Try not to have another accident while you are rushing the cat to the vet!

Further attempts at first aid will almost certainly do more harm than good. Broken or fractured bones need expert treatment. Leave the job to an expert.

Technique for moving injured cats

Moving a cat in great pain is not the easiest thing to do, so be prepared for some problems. A badly hurt or frightened animal may bite or scratch anyone who tries to touch it, including its owner. Do not waste time trying to calm the cat with soothing talk; if it is really hurt, it will not hear you. Just take the necessary precautions against being bitten, and get on with the job.

(i) The cat may be lifted by the scruff of the neck and carried to a car.

(ii) The best way to prevent a cat from biting and scratching you while you are trying to move it is to cover it with a blanket or coat, and then gently lift and carry the whole bundle of cat and coat. With serious injuries, roll the cat on to a coat or blanket and carry it in this improvised sling.

(iii) If there is someone with you, have him hold the injured cat while you drive. If you are alone, place the injured cat on the floor of the car, in the front, on the passenger side.

(iv)   It is better and much faster to get the cat to the vet than to get the vet to the cat. If possible, have someone telephone the vet, so that treatment is ready when you arrive. If you do not know a vet, phone the police and they will tell you where the cat should be taken.

Warmth; no fluids

Try to keep the cat warm when you are taking it to the vet. Do not apply external heat, just cover the animal with a coat or blanket. The idea is to prevent loss of body heat. Do not try to numb the pain by pouring whisky down the cat's throat, or try to counteract the shock with warm milk or water. This is to prevent vomiting if an anaesthetic has to be administered.

---

33   Cat falling into a Hot Bath

This happens more than anyone (except a cat owner) would believe. The cause is a combination of the cat's antipathy to water and its overriding curiosity, as well as the slipperiness of bathtubs. If you run yourself a hot bath and if puss can get into the bathroom, then sooner or later . . . Splash!

Treatment

(i)   If the cat has not jumped out by itself, grab a towel and use it to pull the cat out of the bath. With the cat still wrapped in the towel, plunge it into a sinkful of cold water or wrap it in cold wet towels. The object is to reduce the temperature of the body tissues as quickly as you can.

(ii)   If the cat is in a state of shock – indicated by its being semi-conscious or unconscious, by pallor of the mucous membranes, shallow breathing, etc. – then administer half a cup of cooled, strong black coffee. See **Force-Feeding**. Keep the cat wrapped up warmly after you have cooled its burnt tissues, and let it rest.

(iii)   Any breaks in the skin which appear after the cat's bathtub experience should be treated as scalds (moist burns). See **Burns and Scalds.**

(iv)   Half a Paracetamol tablet may be administered if the cat is in pain. See **Tablets and Pills: Techniques of Administration.**

(v)   Wait a few hours before giving the cat any food or water.

All cats are susceptible to cat flu, but the exotic breeds (Siamese, Burmese, Abyssinian, Rex, etc.) are particularly susceptible and in very severe cases may die, despite the most rigorous treatment.

There is no effective vaccine available.

Cat flu cannot be transmitted to human beings or to other species of animal, just to other cats.

Symptoms
The incubation period is from two to four days, and during this period the following symptoms may be observed:

1   The onset of the infection is marked by *temperature above normal* and by sneezing which may be accompanied by excessive salivation (dribbling) and by lethargy.

2   The cat's temperature will continue to rise to about 105°F (40°C) and then fluctuate between this high figure and normal for the course of the disease, which lasts up to three weeks.

3   The next stage is marked by a discharge from the eyes and nose. At first this discharge is clear, but after a day or so it becomes yellow and sticky and particularly noticeable on the chest and on the paws, where the animal has tried to rub the stickiness away. At this stage, in addition to the yellow sticky discharge, the cat loses its appetite.

4   During the course of cat flu, there is progressive dehydration and raw sores appear on the tongue and in the mouth.

Even after a satisfactory recovery, the cat may be left with a chronic infection of the nasal sinuses which causes a yellowy, mucous discharge from its nose.

Home treatment
Cat flu is a virus infection and since viruses do not respond to antibiotics, there is no simple cure for the disease. The cat owner can only treat the symptoms as they arise.

Obviously a vet must be consulted, but correct supportive home treatment is also very important.

(i)   Bathe the cat's eyes and nose with warm water to remove the accumulating discharge.

(ii)   To prevent dehydration and starvation, administer, by force if necessary, glucose and water (up to $\frac{1}{4}$ pint (125 ml) per day) and meat extracts such as Brands Essence (up to $\frac{1}{4}$ pint or 125 ml).

35   Cat up a Tree

A cat sitting on a branch twenty feet off the ground, miaowing piteously, is perhaps a classic example of a potential first aid hazard.

Of course, it is not the cat which is in danger, but rather the anxious cat lover who tries too hard to rescue kitty.

Correct technique
(i)   If a dog has chased the cat up the tree, chase the dog away.
(ii)   Get a tin of cat food, or some fish, and place it at the foot of the tree.
(iii)   Go home and relax, secure in the knowledge that sooner or later the cat will come down.
(iv)   It will come down the same way it went up. Even if it seems impossible to you, be assured the cat will manage to climb down somehow. After all, have you ever seen a dead cat in a tree?

36   Cataracts

A cataract is an opacity and hardening of the lens of the eye, which prevents the light from passing through it.

Causes
1   The most common cause of cataracts is old age. But it must be remembered that cataracts cause varying degrees of blindness. In an elderly cat, the lens may appear quite opaque and yet a certain amount of vision is still possible.
2   If cataracts appear in the eyes of young cats, a disease state, such as diabetes, must be considered.

Symptoms
1   A gradual, growing opacity, or milkiness, of the pupil.
2   The cataract itself resembles a white marble, *inside* the eye and not on the surface of the eye.

Treatment
Cataracts, like every serious eye condition, must be treated by a professional. This treatment should be started as soon as the cat owner notices the cloudiness. Delay can prevent possible cure.

In many cases a non-functional lens can be removed surgically, resulting in the return of a fair degree of vision.

37　Choking

Choking takes place when either the tongue or a foreign body blocks the back of the throat and prevents the cat from breathing. Choking often looks and sounds much worse than it really is because the cat panics, which makes it choke even more, which makes it panic even more . . . *Don't you panic, too.*

Treatment
If the cat has passed out (from lack of oxygen), open its mouth and pull its tongue out; make certain that nothing is blocking the windpipe. If there is something blocking it, do not try to push whatever it is down the cat's throat. Hook it out with your finger. Once the throat is clear, if the cat is still unconscious, artificial respiration should be given. See **Artificial Respiration.**
If the cat is conscious, hold it upside down, by its hind legs, and thump it on the back. This may dislodge whatever is down its throat. If it does not, and the cat is still choking, open its mouth (see **Opening a Cat's Mouth**), and use your fingers to fish out the foreign object. If the object is stuck, pour a little olive oil down the cat's throat to lubricate the gullet. If your probing causes the cat to gag, so much the better, as this may bring up the obstruction.

38　Clipping Nails

Cats which do not get enough exercise may need their claws trimmed. If the claws are long enough to catch on material, it is time to trim, or chance a broken claw.

Technique
If the quick cannot be seen, cut along the line formed by the base of the nail (see illustration 6).

WARNING
Do not clip the nail too short or you will cut the vein under the nail and cause the toe to bleed.
　　Should this happen, the bleeding can be controlled by bandaging the nail (see **Bandaging**), or by applying a styptic pencil to the site of the bleeding.

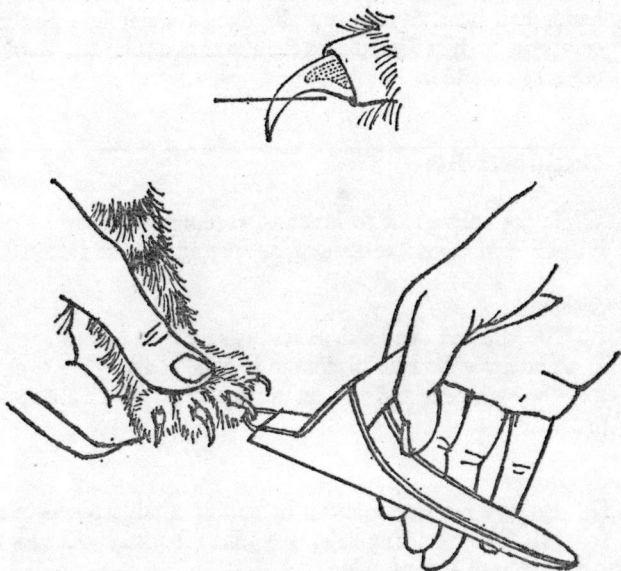

---

39   Colds

Cats do not catch colds. But if a cat exhibits the symptoms of the common cold, do not treat these symptoms lightly. These symptoms suggest something more serious. See **Cat Flu, Pneumonia, Sinusitis.**

---

40   Compresses, Cold and Hot

A compress is made by taking a wad of cotton wool or material and saturating it in the proper solution. Hot and cold compresses may be used in conjunction with each other, e.g. for sprains and strains, use alternate hot and cold compresses.

Cold compresses
Cold compresses or ice packs are applied directly over a swelling which has been caused by concussion, and will bring the swelling down.

Hot compresses

Hot compresses are especially effective for reducing pain. They are made by placing cotton wool in the hottest water your hands can bear. Wring out the excess water and apply the compress to the affected area for about two minutes. Repeat as often as possible.

---

41   Conjunctivitis

While not contagious to humans, conjunctivitis can be transmitted from animal to animal, so quarantine the infected cat.

Symptoms
1   The affected eye reddens and is sore to the touch.
2   A sticky yellowish discharge is exuded from the eye.
3   The eye hurts and the cat continually rubs its face on the ground.

Treatment
(i)   Prepare a saline solution by adding 2 tablespoons iodine-free salt (plain cooking salt) to 1 pint (500 ml) boiling water. Allow to cool before using.
(ii)   Bathe the eye liberally with the solution every two hours for the next twenty-four hours.
(iii)   If the condition does not clear up within thirty-six hours, get professional help. See **Foreign Bodies.**

---

42   Constipation

Causes
Often occurs in cats which are fed bones in their food and in cats with rectal tumours, abdominal tumours, slipped discs and after fractures of the pelvis.

Symptoms
Straining. Passing a brown watery discharge. Possible bleeding from the anus. In some cases, vomiting may occur.

Treatment
Administer 1 tablespoon (25 ml) liquid paraffin (an excellent laxative), and stop feeding the cat bones. If the cat does not have a bowel movement within twenty-four hours of receiving

the laxative, contact a vet. The cause of the constipation may be more serious and an enema may be necessary. If a vet is not available, you will have to administer the enema yourself. See **Enema.**

If constipation is suspected in a cat which usually goes out of doors, it will be necessary to confine the cat to the house, so that its litter tray may be inspected.

---

43   Cough Medicine

A cough medicine is a product designed to soothe or suppress a cough.

Before administering cough medicines or soothing syrups, take into consideration that a cough is not a separate entity, but a possible symptom of many diseases, and treatment of the symptom will not remedy or remove the cause. A cough medicine may stop the cough (temporarily) and allow the cat a rest. However, it will not *cure* whatever is causing the cough.

If possible, try to determine the cause of the cough before administering the cough medicine.

Treatment
(i)   Give 5 ml Diphenhydramine (Benylin) twice a day. Or,
(ii)   try a home-made solution of 2 tablespoons (50 ml) honey in 2 tablespoons (50 ml) water, with 1 teaspoon (5 ml) lemon juice added, to soothe the cat's irritated throat. See **Force-Feeding.**

If, after forty-eight hours, the animal is still coughing, a vet should be consulted.

---

44   Cracked Pads

Symptoms
Cats suffering from cracked pads will be lame on pavements and other hard surfaces but will walk without limping on grass.

Treatment
(i)   Get a good light and examine the paw carefully. Make sure that the trouble is not caused by a cut pad. Also check to be sure that the cat's lameness is not the result of a cracked nail.
(ii)   Treat the simple cracked pad or sore pad by bathing it in a solution of very strong cooled tea (tannic acid) with 4

tablespoons (100 ml) witch-hazel added. The easiest way to bathe the painful paw is to pour the tea into a bowl and then put the cat's foot into the bowl and allow it to soak for a few minutes, or for as long as you can hold the paw in the bowl. Do this twice a day for three days.

(iii)   Then, treat the cracked pad by rubbing it with olive oil, baby oil or with lanolin three times a day for three days.

(iv)   The general rule regarding cut or cracked pads is, if they are not bleeding, the less treatment the better.

---

45   Dandruff (Scurf)

Not uncommon in cats with dry coats. It looks exactly like human dandruff: fine white flakes scattered through the coat, especially along the spine.

Treatment
This is a skin condition, and it should be promptly treated to prevent it from becoming a problem.

Shampoo the cat once a week for four weeks with a selenium-based shampoo such as Selsun. See **Shampooing a Cat.**

Also, give the cat one teaspoon of corn oil daily for one week.

Cats with a tendency towards this dry flaking of the skin should have corn oil added to their diet regularly. One tablespoon (25 ml) corn oil per week should prevent the condition from recurring.

---

46   Deafness

Deafness, unfortunately, is fairly common in cats. It can be either hereditary or acquired.

Hereditary deafness
Usually found in white cats, with blue eyes. Cats suffering from hereditary deafness should be sterilized to prevent them from passing on the condition.

Acquired deafness
Acquired deafness often occurs as the result of ear infections or accidents. It may be irreversible or temporary, depending upon the cause and the severity of the condition.

Partial deafness

Partial deafness occurs in elderly cats, and in younger ones which have ingested poisons containing lead.

Symptoms
1 Deaf cats may appear to be stupid. They do not respond to their names, or to commands, and they are apt to miaow continually.
2 A definite diagnosis of true deafness is difficult, since the deaf cat is compensated by the enhancement of its other sensory perceptions, especially the ability to detect vibrations.

---

47 Death

Eventually, all cats die. The problem is how to be certain that the animal is dead.

Symptoms
1 Immediately after death, the cat's body is limp and flaccid.
2 The eyes are glazed, the pupils dilated. A light shone into the eyes gives back a green reflection.
3 There is complete absence of pulse, heartbeat and breathing.
4 Hold a mirror close to the animal's nose. If the cat is breathing, the mirror will mist over.
5 If the cat is dead, after a few hours its body will stiffen, as *rigor mortis* sets in.
6 Eventually, decay begins.

---

48 Destruction

Animals in their natural wild state rarely die of old age. Having extended the life-span of our cats by protecting them as far as possible from illness and accident, we have the responsibility of caring for them in their old age and finally of sparing them any unnecessary suffering.

A part of that responsibility is the decision as to when that point of unnecessary suffering has been reached. Chronic illness, incontinence, senility are the factors to be balanced against more subjective feelings such as the cat owner's love of his pet and the sanctity of life in general.

C

While the final decision is the individual cat owner's responsibility, too often people permit their old pets to linger on painfully, hoping that the poor old thing will die soon. When you find yourself feeling that way, perhaps it is time to do your cat one last kindness.

When a cat is put down by a veterinary surgeon, the process is simple and painless. The cat is given an injection of an anaesthetic. Before you can count to three, the animal is dead. Its troubles, aches and pains are over.

The most difficult situations arise when a cat has been badly injured, usually in a car accident, and is in great pain. Most people are not equipped to destroy the animal. So, rather than take the chance of causing even greater pain, call the police at once. They will give you the emergency telephone number of the nearest vet. Leave this sad job to him.

49   Diabetes

Diabetes Insipidus (Drinking Diabetes)
Symptoms
1   The cat drinks vasts amounts of water. *Be sure to keep its water bowl full.*
2   There is no smell of acetone on the breath, as in **Diabetes Mellitus** (see below).
3   The cat urinates frequently; the urine is very pale. Laboratory tests show that there is no sugar in the urine. See also **Kidney Failure.**

Treatment
The vet may put your cat on a course of hormone treatment.

Diabetes Mellitus
Cause
Malfunction of the pancreas, leading to an abnormal amount of sugar in the blood. This condition is rare in cats.

Symptoms
1   There is increased thirst and increased urination. A laboratory analysis would show traces of sugar in the blood.
2   There is a marked increase of appetite.
3   There may be loss of weight.
4   There is a sweetish odour of acetone (which smells like nail-polish remover) on the animal's breath.

5 Secondary symptoms of cataracts may appear in the eyes.
6 If untreated, the animal will fall into a diabetic coma. See **Unconsciousness.** A definite diagnosis must be made by a vet, after analysis of a urine sample. See **Taking Samples of Faeces and Urine.**

Treatment
(i) Home treatment after professional consultation may consist of daily injections of insulin. See **Injections.**
(ii) Insulin should always be given *before* feeding.

OVERDOSE
If an accidental overdose of insulin is administered, insulin coma will follow. This condition may be reversed by giving a tablespoon of crushed or powdered sugar. Sprinkle a little at a time into the unconscious cat's mouth.

---

50   Diarrhoea

This is the name given to a condition where loose, unformed faeces are passed. Cats are natural scavengers and often suffer mild attacks of diarrhoea as a result of eating decayed foodstuffs. It can also be the result of an incorrect diet, bacteria, viruses or poison.

Symptoms
1 Frequent passing of loose motions.
2 Foul-smelling motions.
3 The diarrhoea may be associated with vomiting or it may appear on its own.

Treatment
(i) All food and water should be withheld for twenty-four hours.
(ii) After twenty-four hours, give a cupful of water per day and small amounts of boned chicken and rice or fish and rice to eat for the next few days. There are a few finicky cats which, under normal circumstances, will not eat rice, but if hungry enough, a cat should eat just about anything, rice included.
(iii) No milk should be given for one week.
(iv) If the diarrhoea persists, starve the cat again for another twenty-four hours. Then give the following mixture: 3–4 tablespoons glucose powder, 1 raw egg white and 1 pinch

salt mixed into ½ pint (250 ml) warm water. Give the animal 2 tablespoons (50 ml) of this mixture every two hours for two days. See **Force-Feeding**.

(v)   Then put the cat on a diet of chicken and rice or fish and rice for two to three days, before resuming normal feeding.

Persistent Diarrhoea

If the diarrhoea persists for more than forty-eight hours, it may be the symptom of more serious diseases. A vet must be consulted.

Sore Anus

Cats with diarrhoea may develop a sore anus. Apply cold cream or vaseline to help soothe the irritated area.

---

51   Diet

An adequate diet is one which is palatable and which, when fed regularly, will maintain good health without the development of deficiency diseases. However, some cat owners tend to feed their pets on what the animal prefers, or to feed them foods which are convenient to give and/or easy to prepare, without regard for the animal's nutritional requirements. Most cats are accommodating animals: they will eat whatever you give them and will maintain a reasonable nutritional level.

This does not mean that cats can be fed whatever is convenient. Convenience is fine, but a well-balanced diet is essential. A well-balanced diet should contain the correct proportion of proteins, carbohydrates, fats, minerals and vitamins.

The simplest adequate ration for a healthy cat would consist of good quality raw meat containing about 5 per cent fat, with the occasional addition of offal in the form of heart, liver or kidneys.

Cooked, boned fish can be substituted for meat occasionally. Canned foods provide a convenient and totally balanced diet, but in some cases the price may be considered prohibitive. We do not recommend the feeding of dried or soft moist foods exclusively.

Feeding amounts

Four ounces (100 g) per 10 lb (5 kg) body weight per day. This figure is based on the assumption that the cat is getting enough exercise. If, for some reason, this is not the case, the food supply should be reduced proportionately, up to half the normal amount.

Diet for brood queen
A brood queen is a cat which is used for breeding. Brood queens may be fed their usual diet, with extra milk and fat added. About an extra ½ pint (250 ml) milk per day, plus 2 egg yolks, should be adequate.

Also add 2 tablespoons sterilized bone-flour once a week to the queen's food.

Do not feed the queen dried foods from the day of mating until birth occurs. These contain carbohydrates, which tend to make cats fatter, and a pregnant animal should not be overweight.

Feeding times
Cats should be fed regularly at the same hour every day. In this respect they are creatures of habit, and at the accustomed hour their gastric juices begin to flow.

Kittens
Kittens should receive meals as follows:
 at eight weeks, four times a day
 at fourteen weeks, three times a day
 at eighteen weeks, twice a day
 at six months, once a day.

Adult cats
Grown cats may be fed once or twice a day, depending upon the cat's appetite and upon exercise. Elderly cats should be fed two or three smaller meals, rather than one large meal.

---

52 Dislocations

Dislocations occur when a bone has become displaced (pulled away) from the joint. They should not be confused with *fractures*, which are broken bones. Unlike fractures, most dislocations should not be splinted.

Symptoms
1 While a fractured limb tends to swing freely, a dislocated limb is more rigid.

2   There is usually pain and swelling round the dislocated joint and the leg may point in an odd direction, especially in the case of a dislocated elbow.

3   The cat may attempt to walk on the dislocated leg and the leg may support some of the weight before giving way.

Treatment
Do not bandage dislocated limbs. Take the cat to a vet.

Dislocated hip joint
If a dislocated hip cannot be corrected, in four to six weeks a false joint will develop. This will work almost as well as the original.

A false joint is one which is formed as a result of the formation of scar tissue. However, a dislocation must not be left to nature; see a vet at once.

---

53   Drowning

Despite their aversion to water, cats are usually excellent swimmers. However, like human swimmers, they can drown.

Treatment
Get the cat out of the water. Then:
(i)   If the animal is unconscious, lay it on its side and open its mouth. Make sure that its tongue is out and that there is nothing obstructing the windpipe. Use your finger to check for grass, sand, mud, etc in the cat's mouth.
(ii)   If the cat is still unconscious, lift it by its hind legs and allow the water to drain out of its mouth.
(iii)   Administer artificial respiration or mouth-to-mouth respiration, which is slightly more effective (see **Artificial Respiration**).

---

54   Eczema

A common condition in cats. It is a general term for a superficial inflammation of the skin, and occurs in various forms.

Acute eczema
Symptoms
1   Severe itching.

2   The hairs around the affected areas are broken and sparse.
3   The skin around the affected areas is bright red and sore.
In long-haired breeds this may lead to the disease's going
undetected, due to the matting of the animal's coat.

Acute moist eczema
1   Constant scratching.
2   This condition is typified by the sudden appearance of a
large wet area exuding serum. (Serum is a yellowish fluid
which dries to a yellowish crust.) Very painful breaks in the
skin can appear overnight. These lesions are most common
in areas that the animal can scratch or lick most easily, and
they vary in size from a penny upwards.
3   Initially, the breaks in the skin are wet and purulent. Then
they dry to a yellow scab.
4   The pain is obvious. The animal loses its appetite and is
distressed.

Treatment
(i)   Apply a solution of potassium permanganate crystals
(available from chemists) to the area: 1 pinch crystals to 1 pint
(500 ml) water.
(ii)   Wash the cat all over with a shampoo containing Selenium
(e.g. Selsun). See **Shampooing a Cat.**
(iii)   After drying the cat, dab calamine lotion on the affected
areas.
(iv)   If after twenty-four hours the irritation persists, contact
the vet.

Chronic eczema
Causes
1   Usually dietary: excess carbohydrates, fat deficiency,
vitamin deficiency, feeding fish exclusively. Cats are so fond
of fish that they will eat fish and fish only if you permit it.
Make certain that your cat eats a balanced diet. See **Diet.**
2   Allergies.
3   Dirty skin.
4   Abrasions from collars and harnesses.
5   Friction between elbow and chest.
6   Hormonal imbalance.
7   Individual predisposition.

Treatment
Identify the cause and correct it where possible.

Labial eczema
A form of eczema which attacks the lips.

Symptoms
The lips are red and sore, with the surrounding hair on the muzzle becoming brown-stained and foul-smelling.

Treatment
(i)   Clip the hair around the lips with a pair of scissors with rounded ends, the type used for cutting children's finger nails. You will need someone to hold the cat while you do the clipping. See **Restraint.**
(ii)   Wash the area well with soap and water daily.
(iii)   For very severe cases, paint the sore areas with a silver nitrate pencil. Wear rubber gloves or you will burn your fingers. If home treatment is not successful, then professional treatment will be necessary.

Miliary eczema
Cause
This form of eczema is the result of either various hormone deficiencies, or the result of feeding the cat too much fish, to the exclusion of other dietary essentials.

Symptoms
1   There will be severe itching; the owner usually first notices the cat scratching more than usual.
2   Upon examining the cat's fur, the owner will observe – usually on the animal's back, along its spine – small scabs at the base of the hairs.

Treatment
(i)   Stop feeding the cat fish. If you have not been feeding fish, suspect a hormone deficiency and get professional assistance.
(ii)   Bathe the cat with a selenium-based shampoo, e.g. Selsun. Even though the cause may be hormonal, the cat will be scratching itself and its skin should be kept clean. Shampoo once a week for a month. See **Shampooing a Cat.**
(iii)   Administer vitamin C tablets: 50 mg daily.
   If there is no improvement after a week of home treatment, hormone therapy may be required. Seek professional assistance.

55 Electric Shock

Usually caused by the cat's chewing on an electric flex. So, if you find your cat lying flat out next to a badly frayed electric flex, it has suffered an electric shock.

WARNING
Be careful. Very often a shocked cat urinates, and the pool of urine makes an excellent conductor. So do not step on it and do not touch the cat until you have turned off the current, or you will need someone to give **you** first aid!

If you are unable to turn the electricity off, then put on a rubber glove or grab a thick dry towel and pull the electric plug out of the socket. Or, if it is easier, get a wooden stick, such as a broomstick, and push the animal out of the urine and away from the electric flex.

Treatment
If the cat has not regained consciousness by this time, administer artificial respiration. See **Artificial Respiration.**

56 Elizabethan Collar

A most useful device when treating cuts, skin diseases, etc. An Elizabethan collar is a device used to prevent a cat from biting various parts of its anatomy, or from scratching at its face, ears or eyes.

Classically, these collars are prepared from stiff cardboard, but the cat may tear this apart, and we recommend plastic containers such as a child's plastic bucket. All that is necessary is to cut the bottom out of the bucket to a size which the animal's head will go through, then punch four more holes around this one, put the strings through and tie it to the cat's collar or around its neck.

The open end must be sufficiently far away from the nose to prevent licking, and this may present difficulties when feeding time comes. If so, the collar can be removed briefly to allow eating and drinking. Initially, the cat will be very distressed by the collar, but this initial distress will pass, and while the cat will never learn to love the collar, it will learn to live with it.

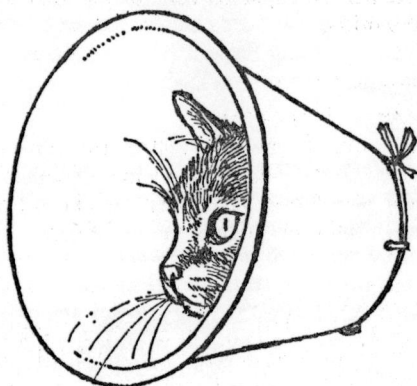

---

57 Emetics (Induced Vomiting)

An emetic is any substance that induces vomiting, and it is usually given after a cat has eaten something poisonous. Table salt is a suitable emetic for cats. If table salt is not available, administer a large crystal of washing soda.

Technique
Take 1 teaspoonful (5 ml) of ordinary table salt or a large crystal of washing soda, and throw it as far back down the animal's throat as possible. See **Opening a Cat's Mouth.**

Obviously, to be effective, the emetic must be administered as soon as possible after the cat has eaten the poison. If the poison has been consumed more than an hour previously, or if the cat is shocked or drowsy, do not induce vomiting.

WARNING
Never attempt to make an unconscious animal vomit.

---

58 Enema

An enema is an injection of non-irritant fluid into the large intestine, administered by way of the anal passage. The purpose of giving an enema is to empty the large intestine of any abnormal or impacted contents, so that the cat can pass a normal motion.

When required
When the cat is constipated.

Enemas may be necessary after the consumption of large amounts of bones (not recommended feeding); or particularly with long-haired cats, after they have been licking their coats and have swallowed large amounts of hair.

How to prepare an enema
The best enema solution is produced by lathering some good-quality soap into a washing-up bowl full of warm water: ¼ pint (125 ml) warm water, with good-quality hand soap or soap flakes that contain no detergents.

This solution is then administered into the rectum via the anus by means of an enema pump.

If a ready-made enema is not available, you can improvise one, using a length of rubber tubing – approximately ⅓ in (1 cm) in diameter – leading to a funnel filled with the enema fluid.

Technique
(i)   Spread some newspapers around the area *before* you give the enema; you will not have time afterwards.
(ii) Have someone hold the cat. Enemas should be given only with the animal standing. See **Restraint.**
(iii) Introduce about 2 in (5 cm) of tubing into the cat's rectum. A little vaseline on the end of the tubing helps.
(iv) Hold the container higher than the cat.

Dosage
Administer 1–3 tablespoons (25–75 ml) of the enema fluid. If the substances that are causing the impaction have not been passed after three attempts, professional help should be sought.

---

59   Excessive Drinking (Drink-Vomit Cycle)

Symptoms
Increased thirst is a symptom of several conditions, all of them serious (see SPECIAL NOTE). Since the average cat owner is not

competent to make a diagnosis, follow these general rules until a vet can examine the cat.

Treatment
Never withhold water from a cat with excessive thirst, unless the cat is vomiting. When a cat starts on the drink-vomit cycle, it will continue drinking and then vomiting until dehydration and death occur.

To break this cycle, withhold all water for twelve hours. Then give the cat 1 tablespoon (25 ml) of a water and glucose mixture, every two hours for twelve hours. The mixture should consist of 3–4 tablespoons glucose powder dissolved in 1 pint (500 ml) water. While cats will not usually drink such a sweet mixture willingly, a cat which has not had a drink for twelve hours will drink almost anything. An ice cube may also be given every hour.

If after twelve hours, the cat is still vomiting, professional help must be sought.

SPECIAL NOTE (differential diagnosis)
Diabetes; chronic interstitial nephritis; pyometritis; increased body temperature; poisoning; enteritis; gastritis; other infections.

These disease states are beyond the scope of home treatment. They are noted here to impress on the cat owner the seriousness of the excessive thirst symptom. A cat exhibiting symptoms of excessive thirst must be carefully observed for a few hours and, if the symptoms are confirmed, professional help must be obtained.

---

60 Eyeball out of Socket

This sometimes occurs after fights or road accidents.

Treatment
(i)   Apply olive oil or vaseline to the eye socket, and gently try to ease the eyeball back into place. Then bandage over.
(ii) If the eyeball will not fit or will not stay in the eye socket, hold the eye in with a pad of damp or oily cotton wool (saturate cotton wool with olive oil).
(iii) Bandage over lightly. See **Bandaging.**
(iv) Seek professional help.

61   Feline Enteritis

A very common and very serious virus infection.

Symptoms
1   Depression and lethargy.
2   Loss of appetite.
3   High temperature – 101.5°F to 106°F. See **Temperature Taking.**
4   Vomiting.
5   Dehydration. To test for dehydration, pinch a bit of the cat's skin between your fingers. If the cat is dehydrated, the skin remains pinched for a few minutes instead of immediately returning to its normal shape.
6   A classic symptom of this disease is the cat sitting hunched over its drinking bowl, but not drinking.

Treatment
If any combination of the above symptoms appears, get professional advice at once. Feline enteritis develops rapidly and can kill a cat within 8 hours from the onset of the initial symptoms.

Prevention
All cats should be vaccinated against feline enteritis. Kittens may be vaccinated any time after twelve weeks of age, with a booster shot once a year. Make sure your cat is vaccinated. See **Vaccination.**

62   First Aid Kit

All animal owners should prepare a first aid kit and keep it in a tin, clearly marked, and in a safe place. It should contain:
  A pair of sharp-edged, blunt-pointed scissors.
  A pair of forceps (tweezers).
  Four rolls of 2 in (5 cm) elastoplast.
  Four rolls of 2 in (5 cm) roller bandage.
  A packet of cotton wool.
  A packet of lint.
  A bottle of 20 vol hydrogen peroxide.
  A bottle of antiseptic, eg Savlon, Dettol, Roccal.
  A razor blade.
  A packet of needles.

Paracetamol tablets.
A packet of cotton buds.
A crystal of washing soda (emetic).
Table salt.
An eyedropper.
A copy of this book.
The address and telephone number of a local vet.

---

63   Fish Hooks

If a cat gets a fish hook caught in its mouth, or anywhere on its body, if it is at all possible, get the poor creature to a vet at once. It is easy enough to remove a fish hook after the cat has had a general anaesthetic. Unfortunately, most fish hook accidents happen in places remote from vets and it may be up to you to remove the hook.

A cat, unlike a dog, does not paw at its throat or mouth if something is caught there. (And that is where puss usually gets the fish hooks caught.) Instead of pawing, cats usually hunch up and keep gulping. Also, a cat that has been hurt is likely to run off and hide. So, with a cat, the first thing to do is to confine the animal. You do this simply by putting a basket or a box with a weight on top of it over the cat while you gather your tools and find an assistant.

One assistant will do; two are better; three assistants are ideal. It is not absolutely imperative to have three helpers, but it is very helpful.

Preparation

In addition to assistants you will need a pair of needle-nosed pincers or wire-cutters, and a sharp knife or razor blade. Boil the knife or razor blade for twenty minutes.

You will also need a thickish towel and two short lengths of rope or two neckties.

Make sure you have a good light to work in. You must be able to see what you are doing.

Operation

When you have everything together and are ready to proceed, roll the cat tightly in the towel, leaving only its head outside.

The drill is for one assistant to hold the cat in the towel, one assistant to knot a necktie around the cat's upper jaw and hold it as steady as possible, while the third assistant prises open the cat's lower jaw and knots the other necktie around it, using the necktie to keep it open.

Now, look carefully at the way the hook is embedded. Think about what you are doing before you do anything.

Do not try to *pull* the hook out. If you do, you will tear a great bloody chunk out of the animal. Determine which way the barb is pointing and push it out through the skin. Use the pincers or wire-clippers to snip off the head of the hook. Then push it out. Push in the opposite direction from where the barb is pointing.

If the hook is embedded in such a way as to prevent you from getting at the head, you will have to use your sharp, sterile knife to make an incision over the area where the head of the hook is embedded. Don't be too squeamish. Your incision will do much less damage than a forceful pull. After you have made the incision, you can use your pincers to snip off the head of the hook.

When the hook is out, clean the wound with soap and water, and disinfect it by pouring a solution of hydrogen peroxide directly on to the wound. (The hydrogen peroxide will bubble and froth; do not be alarmed, this is quite natural.) The wound is now dressed. But do not let your cat go. If it did not run away before, after what it has just suffered, it is sure to run off now. So it is best to keep your cat confined until it seems to trust you again.

---

64   Fits (Convulsions)

Causes

The cause of a fit cannot be diagnosed from the type of fit or by its severity. The fit may be caused by a number of agents, ranging from minor teething fits to serious infections, to poisons such as strychnine.

Symptoms

Fits take several forms, all of them violent and frightening.
1   The fit usually begins with the cat shaking its head.
2   This is followed by champing of the jaws, salivation, in-co-ordination, screaming, and the involuntary passage of urine and faeces.
3   Then the cat may fall on its side and make running movements.
4   The action of the jaws converts the saliva into a viscid

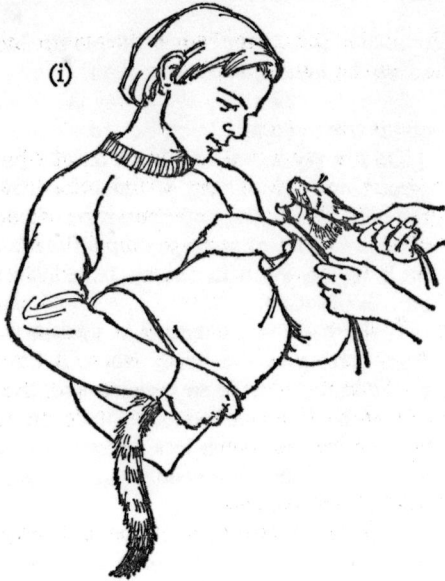

(i)

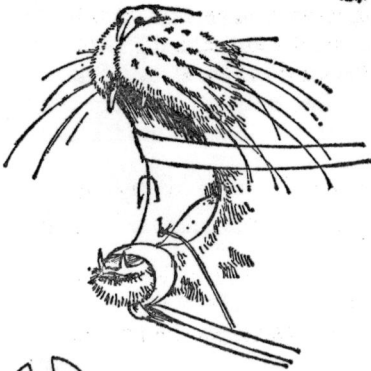

(ii)

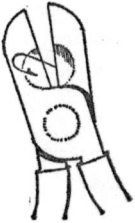

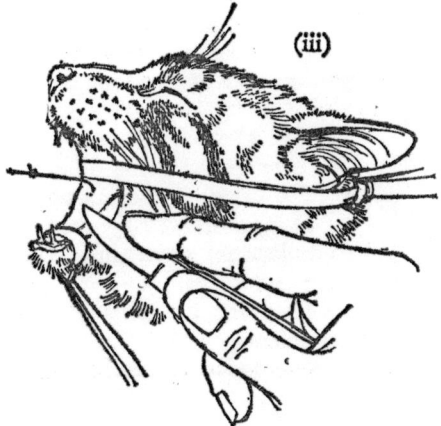

(iii)

froth, causing the cat to foam at the mouth and often terrifying those who should be helping.

Treatment (Immediate)

(i)   The only thing you can do for a cat which is having a fit is to *prevent the animal from hurting itself*. And the first step is to make sure that it does not hurt you. Remember, the most affectionate pet is a dangerous animal during a fit. Do not try to calm it by petting or stroking. It will not do your cat any good. It will just get you bitten or scratched. Do not waste time talking to the cat; it cannot hear you.

(ii)   Move the cat into a place where it cannot injure itself.

(iii)   Get some blankets or pillows and throw them into a closet or small room without furniture or sharp corners. If possible, darken the room.

Technique for moving cats

Throw a blanket or coat over the cat and carry it in this to the room or closet.

Once the cat is in the safe room, leave it alone. The fit will pass. It may take five minutes, it could take thirty minutes, but eventually the fit will pass. When it does, allow the cat to rest quietly.

Further Treatment

Further treatment will depend upon the cause of the fit. Without medical training, one can only make a guess, not a diagnosis.

The fit may have been caused by epilepsy, a virus, by worms, teething, or as the sequel to a very high fever. With very young kittens, it could have been caused by something as simple as overexcitement.

Remember, all you can do is to deal with the immediate situation. Prevent the animal from hurting itself. Further treatment must be left to a vet.

---

65   Fleas

Fleas, like taxes, are a perennial problem for cat owners. Fleas not only cause your cat intense irritation and discomfort, they carry tapeworm eggs, so get rid of them.

Your cat's fleas may bite you, but you will be glad to know that it is only in passing; these fleas will not live on humans.

Description
1 When grooming your cat, if you notice small, reddish, flat creatures running through the fur, your cat has fleas.
2 When the fur of an animal with fleas is parted, it will look as though tiny particles of black grit have been scattered through the hairs. These are flea droppings.

Treatment
(i) Give the cat a bath with a shampoo containing selenium, such as Selsun (available from chemists), every three days for two weeks. See **Shampooing a Cat.**
(ii) When the cat is not being bathed, powder it thoroughly with a patented flea powder containing either pyrethrum or derris powder (available from chemists and most pet shops), once a week.
(iii) During the flea season, which varies from locale to locale, the cat should wear a flea collar (available from pet shops). Change the collar at regular intervals of three to five weeks.
(iv) Supplement baths and powderings with patented aerosol sprays (available from pet shops). These kill fleas on contact.
(v) Dust flea powder around the cat's basket.

Treatment for kittens
Kittens under eight weeks of age should not be powdered. Simply bath them in a solution of selenium shampoo. Make sure that you wash off all the shampoo after bathing. Dry well.

As well as de-fleaing the cat, be sure that the cat's environment, your home, is also free of fleas. To remove fleas from carpets and cushions, spray with any patented aerosol. For heavy infestations, call your local authority.

---

66 Force-Feeding

When it is necessary to force a cat to eat or drink something, the technique is similar to the one used for the administration of tablets and pills.

With Assistant
Hold the Cat
(i) You should have an assistant to hold the cat while you do

the feeding. The assistant holds the cat by the scruff with one hand and wraps his other arm around the animal's back legs. (ii)   Alternatively, the cat is wrapped in a thick towel or blanket, with only its head protruding. The assistant holds the well-wrapped cat tightly.

Open the Cat's Mouth

(iii)   You proceed to open the cat's mouth by placing your left hand on top of the animal's head, with your thumb and index finger placed behind the canine teeth (the fangs). Then firmly pull the cat's head backwards. This will force the mouth open.

Feeding Fluids

(iv)   The food or fluid is administered with the right hand. If it is a fluid, use a plastic spoon, so that if the cat does bite down hard, it won't damage its teeth on metal. With the spoon held in your right hand, slowly pour the liquid as far back in the cat's mouth as possible. The slower you pour the contents of the spoon down the cat's throat, the less chance there is of the cat gagging or choking.

Feeding Solids

(v)   Break the solid food into small, pill-sized bits, and using your right hand, place these bits, one at a time, at the back of the cat's throat. After each bit, hold the cat's jaw shut, until the animal licks its nose. This means the cat has swallowed. Open its mouth and feed it another bit.

(vi)   Flavoured meat extracts may be fed simply by rubbing some on the cat's nose. A cat will lick anything off its nose. This is often a way of stimulating a sluggish appetite. Once a cat gets a taste off its nose, it may begin to eat voluntarily.

Without Assistant

There are easier things than attempting to hold *and* force-feed a cat on your own. But if you must, get everything ready before you begin. Then use your left hand to open the jaws, as described above, and your right hand for spooning in the food.

Some owners can manage this simply by approaching their cat from behind, squatting down and holding the cat between their legs while they get on with the job. Others, force-feeding without an assistant, have to wrap their cat in a towel, with just its head protruding, and then hold the cat by tucking it under their arm. Still others never manage it at all.

67   Foreign Bodies

In the ear
Symptoms
1 Excessive shaking of the head.
2 Scratching of the ear.

Treatment
Most foreign bodies in the ear can be removed by pouring a little olive oil or cooking oil into the ear, then gently massaging the ear until the object is floated out. If the object does not float out, contact a vet. You can judge the urgency of the case by the animal's behaviour.

WARNING
Never poke anything smaller than your left elbow into a cat's ear.

In the eye
The foreign body may be a grass seed, a bit of grit or a grain of sand. In other words, anything which does not belong in the eye is called a 'foreign body'.

If the foreign body punctures the eyeball, it will cause extreme pain. You will probably see the object sticking out of the eyeball. Do not attempt to remove it – get the cat to a vet.

Symptoms
Sudden and profuse crying. But the tears flow out of one eye only. There will be acute irritation of that eyeball as well.

Treatment
Make a saline solution (sterile solution) by adding 1 teaspoon (5 ml) cooking salt to 1 pint (500 ml) boiling water. Allow it to cool.

Bathe the eye liberally with this saline solution. Use an eye-dropper or saturate a wad of cotton wool with the solution and squeeze into the eye.

Apply a soothing ophthalmic ointment (available from chemists) directly on to the eyeball. To do this, place the thumb and index finger of your left hand above and below the affected eye. Squeeze the ointment into the corner of the eye with your right hand. Close the eyelid with the thumb and index finger of your left hand and hold it closed for a few seconds. This will spread the ointment over the whole eyeball.

If, after this treatment, the cat persists in scratching its eye, you may not have flushed out the object. In this case, take the cat to the vet and leave further treatment to him.

In the foot

Foreign bodies in the foot pads are usually pieces of glass which cut the pad and work their way into the paw, or pieces of grit which have found their way into existing breaks.

Symptoms
1 Acute lameness, hobbling.
2 The cat may chew at its foot.
3 In later stages, the affected foot will be hot and swollen and the skin of the pad will be shiny.
4 There may be pus coming from the hole caused by the object.

Treatment
(i) Get the cat into a good light.
(ii) Sterilize a needle by boiling it for twenty minutes, and carefully probe the hole until the foreign object is visible. This will be easier if an assistant holds the cat, wrapped in a towel, with only its head and the affected paw protruding.
(iii) With the aid of tweezers, remove the object. Use the same technique as you would for removing a splinter from your own foot.
(iv) Disinfect by pouring some dilute hydrogen peroxide over the wound, and dress it.
(v) If probing with a needle does not remove the foreign body, prepare a kaolin poultice and apply this to the affected pad for two days. Keep the poultice in place by bandaging it to the cat's foot, and change the poultice and bandage twice a day. See **Bandaging.**
   This should draw the object out, or at least make it easier to remove it with a needle and tweezers.

Kaolin Poultice
Kaolin may be purchased at a chemist. Prepare the poultice by heating the kaolin clay and pouring it on to a wad of cotton wool. Do not apply the poultice if it is too hot. Judge this by applying to the back of your hand. It should be very hot, but not so hot that it burns.

68   Fractures

A fracture is the term used to describe a broken bone.

Simple fracture
If only the bone is broken and there is no communicating wound between the fracture and the skin, it is called a simple fracture.

Compound fracture
If the skin over the fracture site is broken, thus making it possible for germs to enter from the external wound, it is called a compound fracture.

Complicated fracture
This type of fracture may be either simple or compound, but there is also injury to some internal organ, blood vessel, nerve or joint.

Causes
Most fractures are caused by accidents, but occasionally they occur spontaneously, when a bone is undergoing pathological change, such as in a calcium deficiency or bone cancer.

Fractures of the bones of the foot
Symptoms
After a foot injury, if the cat is acutely lame, but the foot not swollen, it is reasonable to assume that the bone is seriously damaged and quite possibly fractured.

Treatment
Place bits of cotton wool between the toes and then wrap a bandage around the leg. Cover the bandage with surgical tape to keep it in position. See **Bandaging.**

Fractures of the jaws
Fractures of the jaws are frequently seen in cats which have fallen from a considerable height. When a cat falls from a height, the front legs sometimes give way and the chin hits the ground, causing a fracture of the lower jaw. In lower jaw fractures, the jaw usually hangs slightly open and there is dribbling from the mouth.

If the cat falls from an even greater height, it may sustain a fracture of the upper jaw, which under close examination appears as a split in the roof of the mouth, which may be accompanied by displacement of the front teeth.

Upper or lower jaw, the difference is mainly academic, since there is no really effective home treatment for this condition. Once you have determined that the cat has a fractured jaw, get the injured animal to a vet without delay.

While many fractures will heal by themselves, there is the very real danger of the jaw healing improperly if no professional treatment is given.

Fractures of the limbs
The fractures most commonly seen in cats are those involving the legs.

Symptoms
1 Acute and profound lameness of the affected leg.
2 Considerable pain.
3 Possible swelling.
4 Possible shortening.
5 When the cat is lifted off the ground, the affected limb will swing freely.

As a general rule, some or all of these symptoms will be seen in a cat with a leg fracture.

General treatment
(i)   Injured cats must be approached and handled with great caution. An animal in pain is dangerous to you and to itself.
(ii)   If a fracture is suspected, handle the limb or broken bone as little as possible.
(iii)   Make the cat as comfortable and as warm as you can. Administer half a Paracetamol tablet to control the pain. See **Tablets and Pills: Techniques of Administration.**
(iv)   Do not attempt to reduce fractures and reset bones in the correct position. This will cause extreme pain and should be done under an anaesthetic.

Lower limbs
These are among the most common fractures seen. The cat will be unable to put its injured foot on the ground and, as it hobbles along, the leg will swing freely. If professional help is not available within twenty-four hours, fractures of the lower leg should be supported by a simple splint. (See below.)

Upper limbs
These are extremely difficult to splint and should be left alone until professional help is available.

To make a splint
You will need an assistant. Have the assistant hold the cat by its scruff with one hand, and with the other hand hold the injured leg on the splint while you tape the leg to the splint.

Lay the cat on its side, injured leg uppermost. Place the injured leg on a thin piece of wood or corrugated cardboard and tape the leg to the wood with strips of elastoplast.

This splint is intended simply to correct excessive movement, as a temporary repair. Get professional aid as soon as possible.

Fractures of the pelvis
Symptoms
A cat with a fractured pelvis will be unable to support any weight on either of its hind legs. However, since a cat with both hind legs fractured, or with a spinal fracture, will also be unable to stand, the only definite way of diagnosing a fractured pelvis is by X-ray.

Treatment
A fracture of the pelvis does not require splinting. Keep the cat in a confined space until a vet has been consulted.

Fractures of the skull
Seen after road accidents, falls, blows. They may cause unconsciousness, nosebleeds and inco-ordination.

Skull fracture can only be diagnosed by X-ray. If a fracture of the skull is suspected, *do not bandage the skull;* it may be a depressed fracture, and bandaging would only make it worse.

If there is bleeding, use simple first aid to stop it. Be very gentle, especially in the area of the skull.

Give no drugs or fluids until a vet has been consulted.

---

69   Frostbite

In this condition, destruction of the tissues is caused by exposure to severe cold. The parts of the body most often frostbitten are the nose, toes, tip of the ears and top of the tail.

Symptoms
1 In mild cases, the frostbitten skin becomes cold and white. There is a loss of hair around the affected areas.
2 In more severe cases, the loss of hair is followed by redness and localized pain.
3 In even more serious cases, the area remains sore, sensitive to the touch, swells, then shrivels. Finally, the skin around the affected area sloughs away, leaving an open weeping surface.

Treatment
(i) In mild cases, increase the circulation of the blood to the frostbitten skin by rubbing the affected area with your hand.
(ii) Then apply a camphorated oil, or oil of wintergreen.
(iii) If the cat is uncomfortable, half of a 300 mg Paracetamol tablet may be administered. See **Tablets and Pills: Techniques of Administration.**
(iv) In the most extreme cases, amputation may be necessary. See **Gangrene.**

---

70   **Gangrene**

The term is applied to either a specific localized condition, or portion of the body in which the tissues are dead because the blood supply to that portion of the body has been restricted.

Infection symptoms
1 When gangrene is due to an infection, it usually follows bite wounds, especially on the feet. *If the infection is left untreated, it may become gangrenous.*
   A bite around the area of the wrist can become infected, causing swelling and pus which block the blood vessels leading to the toes, resulting in gangrene of the toes.
2 The infection develops fairly rapidly, within two or three days, and the infected area becomes swollen, foul-smelling and gives off a bubbly discharge.

Treatment
This condition requires professional assistance.

Blood restriction symptoms
Gangrene caused by restriction of the blood supply to a part of the body is seen when bandages are applied too tightly or when a tourniquet is left on too long. Gangrene then sets in,

affecting the surrounding area. It also occurs (too frequently) when children put elastic bands around the cat's neck, paws, or scrotum.

Treatment
(i)   Remove the source of constriction.
(ii)   Clean the area with peroxide, Savlon or just soap and water, and apply warm compresses to encourage circulation.
(iii)   Get professional help.

---

71   Gastroenteritis

Gastroenteritis is a general term for an infection of the stomach and the intestines which is characterized by vomiting and diarrhoea.

Symptoms
Fever stage
The cat loses its appetite, mopes about and shows no enthusiasm.

The animal may also run a high fever and may show signs of abdominal pain. Cats with abdominal pain often lie with their rear legs up and their front legs extended. They tend to seek cold places to lie on, and they become restless.

A cat with a high fever will have dull eyes, a dry hot nose, a dull coat. Quite simply, the cat looks ill.

Vomiting stage
The next stage is characterized by continual vomiting. Initially, the vomit is white and frothy. Then it becomes yellow. And in advanced stages, it may become bloodstained. During this vomiting stage the cat will be very thirsty. It will drink and then vomit, setting up a drink-vomit cycle.

Diarrhoea stage
Once the vomiting stage has been established, diarrhoea usually begins. About twenty-four hours later, the diarrhoea becomes bloodstained.

Treatment
Withhold food and water for twenty-four hours. Under no circumstances give milk. If the condition persists, seek professional help.

72   Gingivitis

Gingivitis is an infection of the gums which appears at the margin of tooth and gum. It is often seen in association with tartar.

Symptoms
1   The classic symptom is a red line along the gum, above the tooth or teeth.
2   Halitosis.

Treatment
(i)   Since gingivitis is often caused by general infections of the mouth and throat, as well as by more specific infections, the exact cause of the condition must be identified and eliminated.
(ii)   The gingivitis itself is easily treated by applying a solution made from 20 vol hydrogen peroxide (obtainable from chemists). Use 1 part hydrogen peroxide to 3 parts water.
(iii)   Swab the gums with this solution every three hours (see **Opening a Cat's Mouth**). If the condition has not cleared up after three days of treatment, professional help should be sought.

73   Glucose

A quick energy source to be given when the animal is weak and apathetic. Mix 2–3 tablespoons glucose powder with 1 pint (500 ml) water, or mix the powder in with food.

If glucose powder is not available, a substitute mixture can be made by adding 2 tablespoons sugar to 1 pint (500 ml) water and stirring until the sugar has dissolved.

74   Grass Seeds

In the summer and early autumn, drying seeds of barley grasses can cause a good deal of pain by penetrating between the cat's toes, down its ears, in its eyes. If left untreated, the seeds, which are barbed like fish hooks, will migrate inwards, eventually producing discharging wounds.

In ears
Symptoms
A grass seed down the ear will cause very painful symptoms. The cat will rub its face on the ground, paw at its ears and walk with its head on one side as if trying to dislodge something.

Treatment
Pour warm olive oil or cooking oil into the ear and massage gently to float the seeds out.

In eyes
Symptoms
Profuse crying from one eye only. Extreme irritation of the eye. It will become very red and obviously painful.

Treatment
If the seed has not penetrated the eyeball, wash it out of the eye with a saline solution (see **Saline Solution**). If it has penetrated the eyeball, do not attempt to remove it; get the cat to a vet. Determining whether or not the seed has penetrated the eyeball is a matter of observation. The first rule is to take a good look at whatever you are trying to diagnose or treat. In this case, with the aid of an electric torch, you will be able to see if there is something sticking out of the cat's eyeball.

Between the toes
Symptoms
A grass seed lodged between the toes produces pustules which may cause the cat to limp. If left untreated, the seed will work its way into the foot, producing breaks in the skin.

Treatment
If you can see the seed, use a pair of tweezers to pull it out.

---

75   Grooming

Most cats will groom themselves, but the wise cat owner does not leave the job entirely to the animal. The act of grooming not only helps the cat keep clean, it establishes a physical rapport between cat and owner. This rapport will stand the owner in good stead on those occasions when it is necessary to handle the cat in order to administer first aid.

Healthy cats will do their best to keep their coats clean, but even the most industrious cat is unable to keep up with the accumulation of grime in a city environment. It is well to remember that our cats live in a world six inches to two feet (15-60 cm) in height, about level with car exhaust-pipes.

WARNING
If the cat's grooming is neglected, and its coat is allowed to become filthy and matted, the cat will develop a predisposition for skin diseases.

Grooming of sick animals

(i)   The importance of grooming as a factor in nursing, contributing to the cat's well-being, cannot be overemphasized. Sick cats may neglect their grooming. Sick cats have an excuse; their owners do not.

(ii)   Apart from the fur, keep the eyes, nose, ears and around the mouth clean by wiping them regularly with a little diluted Cetavlon, on cotton wool.

(iii)   A cat with diarrhoea will develop a sore anus. Treat this soreness by applying petroleum jelly, or zinc and castor oil cream (available from chemists) to the irritated area.

Cats resist water most strenuously and, except for special situations, need not be bathed in water. There are several 'dry bath' preparations which will do as well. These are in the form of powder which is dusted into the cat's fur and then brushed out.

All cats should be brushed daily. Long-haired cats should also be combed, and any knots of tangled fur that do not comb out should be cut out with scissors.

Cats which are not brushed regularly develop hair balls in their stomachs, from the accumulation of loose hairs they swallow while grooming themselves (see **Hair Balls**).

---

76   Haemorrhage from the Ear

Often seen after fights or road accidents. Bleeding may be from the ear flap or from inside the ear.

Treatment
Whether the bleeding originates from the ear flap or from the ear itself, the treatment is the same: pack the ear canal with

cotton wool (not too much, just enough to fill the ear without overpacking) and hold this in place.

WARNING
If left untreated, this condition can develop into a middle ear infection.

---

77   Haemorrhage from the Vagina

While very slight bleeding from the vagina can occur during heat periods, heavy bleeding requires the immediate assistance of a vet.

Treatment
(i)   See **Abortion or Miscarriage; Shock.**
(ii)   Keep the queen warm and quiet until professional help is available.

---

78   Hair Balls

Cause
Hair balls usually occur in long-haired breeds which are not being adequately groomed. When the cat licks itself, it swallows those loose hairs which have not been brushed and combed out of its coat. In most instances, these hairs are vomited up; but if this does not happen, then the hairs accumulate in the cat's stomach.

Symptoms
1   Sporadic vomiting.
2   Straining to pass faeces.
3   Occasional constipation.

Treatment
In most cases, the cat will eventually pass the hair ball. In acute cases, where there is continual vomiting after eating, administer 2 tablespoons (50 ml) liquid paraffin. See **Force-Feeding.**

Prevention
(i)   The best method of prevention is the most obvious one: brush and comb your pet regularly. See **Grooming.**

(ii) As a further prevention with cats of long-haired breeds, continue to administer 1 tablespoon (25 ml) liquid paraffin once a week.

---

79   Hair Loss (Moulting)

A certain degree of moulting is natural, occurring twice a year, during the spring and autumn. If the cat loses large amounts of hair at other times, check first to make sure that the animal is being properly groomed. If regular grooming has been carried out, then this loss of hair should be considered abnormal. However, this moulting pattern is altered in cats living in centrally heated environments.

Causes
Excessive hair loss may be due to a thyroid deficiency; chronic nephritis; malnutrition; hormone deficiency; fatty acid deficiency.

With cats, this loss of hair may also be caused by fear, since cats when frightened shed their hair.

Treatment
If this excessive moulting is not caused by a specific disease, then:
(i) Bath and groom the cat. Use a selenium-based shampoo, such as Selsun.
(ii) Add 1 teaspoon (5 ml) corn oil to the moulting cat's diet each week.

---

80   Heat Periods (Oestrus Cycle)

The breeding season occurs twice a year, usually in spring and autumn, and lasts for about four weeks. During these weeks, the queen comes into heat several times, each heat lasting for five to ten days.

The first heat period occurs when the queen is six to fifteen months old. After giving birth, the first heat usually occurs within four to five weeks.

Symptoms
A cat in heat presents a most distressing sight to the inexperienced owner. The queen will roll about on the floor, her

hindquarters raised. She will yowl loudly and persistently and perform pedalling movements with her back legs.

Treatment
A male cat, or a set of earplugs (for yourself). If you do not want kittens, keep the queen indoors during her heat. She is not in agony: she just looks as if she is.

81   Heat Stroke

Cause
Prolonged exposure to a source of heat, or overcrowding. The classic cases of heat stroke are seen when cats are packed into travelling cages which are too small for them, and are improperly ventilated.

Heat stroke is more common in cats with heavy coats. And, of course, the condition is aggravated by lack of water.

Symptoms
Panting, dullness, stumbling, sweating through the foot pads. In the later stages, the cat runs a very high temperature, up to 110°F (43°C), falls into a coma and finally dies.

Treatment
(i)   Give the cat water *immediately*.
(ii)   Cool the cat by hosing and sponging it with cold water and by applying ice packs all over its body, with special attention to the head and chest.
(iii)   Give the cat a drinking bowl full of water, with a tablespoon of glucose mixed into it, and then allow the animal time to drink and rest.

82   Hernia

A hernia is a protrusion of internal tissues through a natural opening, such as the navel, which would normally close in the course of growth. There are four types of hernia: inguinal, scrotal, traumatic and umbilical.

Inguinal hernia
Symptoms
This form of hernia is more common in females. Most queens

have tiny inguinal hernias which never require surgery. When treatment is required, there is a swelling in the groin which, if left, will continue to grow.

Treatment
Surgical.

Scrotal hernia
Symptoms
This form, which occurs only in tom cats, is the equivalent of the female's inguinal hernia. In this form there is a swelling in the scrotum, usually on the right side. This swelling is particularly noticeable after the cat has eaten a heavy meal. There may be discomfort and, in severe cases, acute pain and possible strangulation of the bowel. This occurs when the bowel pushes its way through the herniated hole and becomes compressed, twisted or squashed.

Treatment
The only remedy for this form is surgical.
When diagnosing scrotal hernia, be careful not to confuse it with an abscess. Both appear as swellings, but an abscess will be hot and painful to the touch.

EMERGENCY
If the pain is obviously acute, professional assistance must be sought without delay. The danger comes from possible strangulation of the bowel, and this constitutes an emergency.

Traumatic hernia
Symptoms
Occurs after accidents and manifests itself as a fluctuating swelling, usually on the abdomen. This is really a rupture, and not a true hernia.

Umbilical hernia
Symptoms
Seen fairly frequently in kittens. There is a small protrusion, about $\frac{1}{4}$ inch ($\frac{1}{2}$ cm) long, of the intestinal fat, visible at the navel.

Treatment
This form of hernia is not often serious, provided that the portion of tissue protruding is small, $\frac{1}{4}$ in ($\frac{1}{2}$ cm) or

less. As the kitten grows, the protrusion remains small. So leave it alone.

If the protruding portion is longer than $\frac{1}{2}$ in (1 cm), the kitten should be taken to a vet for some minor surgery.

83 Hiccups

Causes
Kittens which bolt their food often get hiccups. They also get hiccups if their stomachs are empty.

Occasionally, adult cats will also develop hiccups.

Treatment for adult cats
The condition is not serious and usually disappears of its own accord. However, if the hiccups do persist for more than half an hour, administer 1 tablespoon (25 ml) milk of magnesia.

Kittens
There is no need to worry about hiccups in kittens. If the hiccups appear to be causing the kitten distress, put a little olive oil on your finger and gently rub the kitten's abdomen to induce burping.

84 Human Beings bitten by Cats

Treatment
(i)   Wash the bite with soap and cooled boiled water.
(ii) Rinse the soap off.
(iii) Cover the bite with a clean bandage.
(iv) Visit your doctor, or the casualty department of the local hospital. Remember, all animal bites are contaminated and, if it is a deep bite, an anti-tetanus injection should be given.

85 Inability to give Milk (Agalactia)

Agalactia is the inability of the mother cat to give milk.

Causes
The cause can be hereditary; it can be the result of a hormonal

imbalance; or the sequel to an infection or breast cancer.

Agalactia often occurs in cats giving birth to their first litter, especially in oriental breeds.

Symptoms

The behaviour of the kittens is your best indication of agalactia. If the kittens are not getting their milk, they will be restless and fretful, just as a human baby would be. The mother, however, will appear quite normal.

Treatment

(i) Apply warm compresses to the mother's mammary glands for ten minutes at a time, four or five times a day.

(ii) Gentle massage of the mammary glands with olive oil may stimulate and restore their function.

(iii) Hormone therapy with pituitary hormones. This treatment, which requires the services of a vet, may induce milk production within twenty-four hours.

(iv) Treatment of agalactia, of course, applies only to the mother. Meanwhile, the new-born kittens, waiting for the production of milk, must be fed every two hours. See **Orphan Kittens.**

---

86 Inflammation of the Tongue (Glossitis)

Causes

Numerous, most of them serious. The inflammation could be the result of chronic interstitial nephritis, cat flu, corrosive poisons, fish hook wounds, or other trauma.

Symptoms

1 Severe dribbling, accompanied by loss of appetite and halitosis.

2 Raw, red, sore, circular patches. These are ulcers on the tongue.

3 In the later stages, there is a foul brownish drainage from the corners of the mouth, which drips down the chest and paws. Look for drainage stains on the cat's chest and paws.

Treatment

(i) The cat's mouth must be kept as clean as possible by washing it out with a solution of dilute peroxide and very dilute Savlon.

(ii) The solution is made by mixing 1 teaspoon (5 ml) Savlon with 1 pint (500 ml) water, or 1 teaspoon (5 ml) 20 vol peroxide (available from any chemist) with 3 teaspoons (15 ml) water. This solution should be administered every 2 hours for twenty-four hours.

(iii) If, after twenty-four hours, the inflammation has not cleared up, seek professional advice.

---

87   Injections

While it is not usual for cat owners to administer injections, there are occasional situations, such as diabetes or certain long courses of antibiotic treatment, when knowledge of the technique can be very useful.

The subcutaneous injection is an injection *under the skin*, as opposed to the intravenous injection which is an injection directly *into the vein*. Subcutaneous injections are relatively simple to administer and, when properly administered, are completely painless. Medications requiring intravenous injections are beyond the scope of home treatment. When administering an injection, act with confidence and self-assurance. If you are hesitant and unsure of yourself, the cat will sense it and the process will be that much more difficult.

Technique
(i) If there is someone available, ask him to hold the cat for you. See **Restraint**.

(ii) If the cat looks as though it is getting ready to scratch, hold it firmly by the scruff of the neck. Some cat owners feel that gloves and a heavy coat are useful safety measures, but if the cat is properly scruffed and restrained, these are unnecessary encumbrances.

(iii) Saturate a pad of cotton wool with alcohol and swab the skin around the scruff of the neck, where the injection will be administered. Do not make a great production out of this, or you will alarm the cat. A quick rub with the cotton wool is sufficient.

(iv) After filling the syringe, hold it point uppermost and slowly press the plunger until all the air is out of the syringe.

(v) Hold the syringe at the base, between your index finger and thumb. With your other hand, lift a fold of skin at the scruff of the neck into a cone, and slip the needle under the skin below the cone. Press the plunger. Keep the needle as

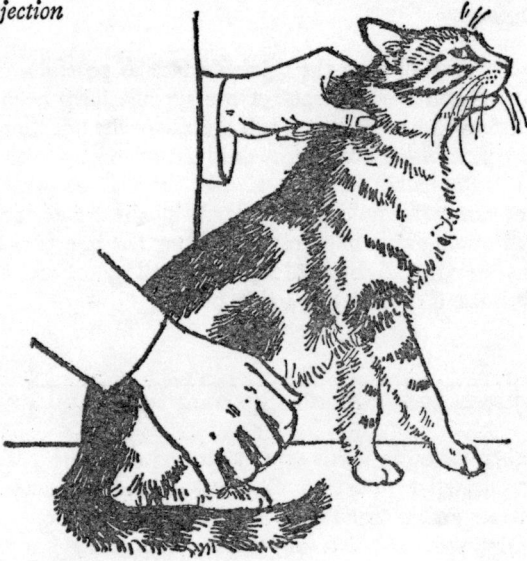

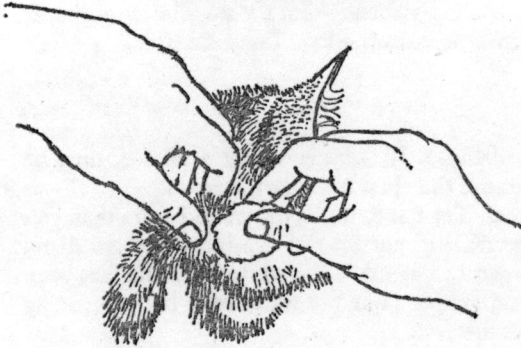

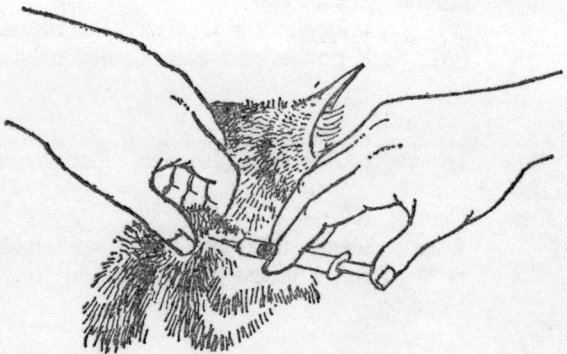

nearly parallel with the skin's surface as possible.

(vi) When the contents of the syringe have been injected, withdraw the syringe and rub the site of the injection for a few seconds to make certain the fluid has been dispersed.

If an assistant is not available, there is no great problem. You can easily hold most animals by the scruff of their neck with one hand, while you administer the injection with your other hand. And, by holding the animal by the scruff, you also minimize the danger of being bitten.

88   Injuries to the Abdomen with Intestinal Protrusion

Cats involved in fights or a variety of accidents (*car accidents*, jumping on to fences, etc) may tear their abdominal wall to such an extent that the internal organs protrude.

Obviously, this is a very serious emergency, but it need not be fatal. The real danger comes from the possibility of shock, or from accidental self-mutilation. Immediate first aid can prevent this.

Treatment
(i)   Assess the damage. If there is no vet available, then be prepared to do more than just bandage the wound.
(ii)   Calm the cat. Try not to touch the wound more than you must. If the protruding portions of the intestines are dirty, they should be gently washed in boiled water, which has been cooled. To wash, simply pour the water over the protruding part of the intestines.
(iii)   If just a small portion protrudes, *gently* try to push it back into the cat's abdomen through the wound.
(iv)   Place a pad over the wound and then bandage the pad around the cat's body.
(v)   Treat for shock if necessary. See **Shock.**
(vi)   Seek professional help immediately.

89   Internal Bleeding (Internal Haemorrhage)

Causes
Road accidents; falls; and eating anticoagulant poisons (such as Warfarin, a mouse and rat poison) can produce internal bleeding.

Symptoms

The overall symptoms are the same as those in cases of severe shock.

1 The cat exhibits pronounced weakness and heavy panting.
2 The pulse rate is very fast (140 plus), but weak. See **Pulse Taking.**
3 The mucous membranes around the lips and nose are pale.
4 The cat's paws will be cold.

Treatment

There is no first aid treatment for this condition. The only certain way of controlling the bleeding is surgical.

EMERGENCY

If these symptoms are observed, *do not waste time*. Wrap the cat in a blanket and get it to a vet. Have someone telephone the vet first, if possible, so that he can have the necessary preparations ready for you when you arrive with the injured animal.

---

90 **Kidney Failure, Renal Failure (Chronic Interstitial Nephritis)**

The disease occurs in two forms. In the first, called the 'compensated form', the cat drinks excessively and is able to flush the poisons through its kidneys. In the second, called the 'decompensated form', the cat is unable to flush the poisons out of its body and may die from the accumulated poisons.

The condition is frequently seen in elderly cats (seven years or older).

Symptoms

The cat is constantly thirsty, and begins to pass more urine, which is pale and watery. The animal's breath is bad.

Its physical condition deteriorates. Its coat is dull and there are skin eruptions. As the condition progresses, the animal vomits frequently and suffers from diarrhoea and excessive urination and thirst.

Treatment

(i) The cat must be given as much clean water as it can drink. Make sure that its drinking bowl is always full.
(ii) Put the cat on a low protein diet of the white meat from

boned chicken or fish, or on a proprietary nephritis diet, available from vets and at most pet shops.

(iii) Antibiotic treatment may be helpful, but this must be left to the discretion of a vet.

---

91 Lameness

See also **Limping**.

In cases of severe lameness, the cat owner should not rely upon his own diagnosis if professional help is available. Improperly diagnosed fractures and dislocations can lead to severe complications.

As a general rule, in diagnosing causes of sudden lameness:
1 If the cat is severely lame and the limb is free-swinging, then the leg is probably fractured.
2 If there is displacement, that is, if the leg is not in its usual position, the leg may be dislocated.
3 If the affected limb is neither free-swinging nor displaced, a strain or sprain or a bite should be suspected.
4 Suspect a foreign body in the pad, or a cut in the pad.

More gradual and more permanent forms of lameness may be encountered with the elderly cat, caused by arthritis or neoplasms (cancerous growths). In such cases, a simple analgesic such as half a 250 mg Paracetamol tablet may help. Do not repeat dosage more than once every forty-eight hours. If the lameness persists for more than a few days, a vet must be consulted. It may be possible to cure the condition by surgical treatment, or, if the condition is non-operative, stronger pain-killers may be indicated.

---

92 Lice

Even though animal lice will not live on human beings, they carry disease and cause intense irritation which may lead to complications. They should therefore be destroyed.

Description
Lice are flat little reddish-brown or black creatures, sometimes confused with fleas. But fleas can be seen running and jumping through the cat's fur, while lice will crawl slowly through the fur, or cling to the base of the hairs.

Treatment
Shampoo and bath the cat twice a week for two weeks with a shampoo containing selenium (Selsun).

---

93   Lightning Strike

Cats sheltering under trees or in close contact with metallic objects, are occasionally struck by lightning.

Symptoms
1   The cat may be burned.
2   The cat may also show signs of shock, such as inco-ordination or even paralysis.

Treatment
(i)   Treat for shock. See **Shock.**
(ii)   Treat the burns. See **Burns and Scalds.**
(iii)   Administer simple stimulants such as strong cooled tea or black coffee. Administer up to 1 cup of either. Hold the cat in a semi-upright position and pour the fluid down its throat slowly, a little at a time, to prevent it from choking.

---

94   Limping

Causes
There are several possible causes for a cat's limping. If the cause is in the foot, the cat may lick the offending paw.

Examine the paw
The first thing to do is to get the cat into a good light and then carefully examine the paw for thorns, tacks or small cuts. You will find that it is easier to do this when the paw is wet, as the hairs lie flat and the thorn or cut is more readily seen.

If it is not a thorn or cut that is causing the limp, look for a cracked pad. You may not be able to see the cracks, so gently palpate the pad with your thumb. A cracked pad is very sensitive and pressure is painful. Be prepared for the cat's reaction.

It is helpful to have an assistant hold the cat while you make the examination. If you are alone, wrap the cat in a towel, with the head and the affected leg protruding.

Next, check for a broken claw-nail or a foreign body (splinter, glass, bit of grit) in the paw. If none of these is evident, the limp may be the result of a sprain or a bite. If it is a sprain, there will be pain and you will be able to feel the local heat. Swelling occurs two to three hours after the sprain or bite. If the limp is caused by a bite, you may find a small puncture wound at the site.

In an older cat, if there is no evidence of a sprain or an injury to the paw, then the limp may be caused by arthritis.

To decide whether or not it is arthritis, observe the cat for a few days, noting:

1 Does the cat have difficulty in rising in the morning? Does it move more easily later in the day?
2 Does a change in the weather bring a variation in the lameness?
3 Is the cat unable to jump up, or manage stairs?
4 Is it lame at a walk? At a gallop?
5 Is the lameness worse with exercise?
6 Is the lameness intermittent?

Treatment
An arthritic condition is not an emergency. However, a cat which limps continually must be seen by a vet. The preceding questions are asked in order to assist the vet in making his diagnosis. If you cannot cure the lameness yourself and you have to take the cat to a vet, these are the questions he will ask you. You should be able to answer them.

As a broad rule of thumb, if the answer to questions 1, 2 and 3 is Yes, then the cat is probably suffering from arthritis. If the answer to questions 4, 5 and 6 is Yes, then the cause of the limping is probably traumatic; that is, the limp has been caused by an accident such as a sprain, cut, blow or bite.

---

95 Mange

Mange is a common skin disease caused by microscopic spider-like creatures. Cats are susceptible to four types of mange. In the order of their frequency, these are: Otodectic mange (ear mite infestation), Notoedric mange, Demodectic mange, Sarcoptic mange.

Otodectic mange
Symptoms
1 Usually, the first symptom observed is a nasty brown

waxy discharge containing brown crusts, in and around the ears.

2 There is acute irritation of the ears, and the cat spends a good deal of time scratching its ears and shaking its head.

3 There may be a rattling noise from the ears when the cat shakes its head.

Treatment

Once again, an assistant is helpful, but not absolutely essential. The first step is to clean the cat's ears. Wrap the cat in a towel with just its head protruding. Clean its ears with cotton wool dipped in a small amount of a very dilute mixture of washing-up liquid: 1 teaspoon (5 ml) washing-up liquid per ¼ pint (125 ml) water. This will get rid of the sticky wax.

Be careful, of course, when you are cleaning the cat's ears, but you need not be afraid of touching the eardrum, since it is well out of the way of cotton wool. Do not use a cotton bud or Q-tip as this may damage the eardrum.

After cleaning, swab the inside of the ear with olive oil or liquid paraffin twice a day for one week.

When treating the cat, use the oil sparingly. Hold the ear flaps while applying the solution. This stops the animal shaking its head.

Notoedric mange

Symptoms

1 Breaks in the skin will appear on the cat's ears and face.

2 There is a marked loss of hair. Bald patches, with greyish-yellow crusts, will be observed.

3 The animal will constantly scratch itself.

4 The skin around the affected area will redden and eventually wrinkle.

Notoedric mange is easily confused with dermatitis, ringworm and demodectic and sarcoptic mange. A definite diagnosis can be made only after a microscopic examination of skin scrapings.

Treatment

Apply sulphur and lime washes, rotenone or sulphur ointments (all available without prescription), by dipping a cotton swab or Q-tip into the ointment and rubbing it gently into the infected areas, for one minute, twice a day. It is also useful to shampoo with a selenium shampoo, e.g. Selsun, every three days for two weeks.

Demodectic mange
This type of mange is quite rare in cats. Its visible symptoms and treatment are the same as those for notoedric mange.

Sarcoptic mange
Symptoms and treatment as above, but this form of mange can affect the cat's entire body. In addition, sarcoptic mange can be transmitted from cats to human beings. Strict sanitary precautions should be taken.

Sanitary precautions
(i)   Throw away any bedding used by the cat.
(ii)   Remove the cat's collar or harness for as long as the condition persists. When you have cured the mange, replace the old collar or harness with a new one.
(iii)   Do not allow the cat to come into contact with other animals. Keep the cat indoors.
(iv)   After every treatment, use liberal amounts of soap and water and Cetavlon to thoroughly clean and disinfect the area where you have been treating the cat. Make certain that you dispose of the cotton wool where no one will touch it.
(v)   Wash your hands.

Relief from excessive biting and scratching
Excessive biting and scratching of the infected areas can cause secondary infections and other complications, so if the poor cat simply will not stop scratching, fit it with an Elizabethan collar. See **Elizabethan Collar.**

You may also provide temporary relief by applying a soothing, cooling lotion, such as calamine lotion, to the irritated areas.

WARNING
Never use carbolic soap or lysol to wash your cat. Cats absorb the carbolic and lysol through their skins, and though these preparations will kill the cat's mange, they may also kill the cat. Also avoid using any soaps or preparations containing coal or wood tar derivatives.

96   Mating (Queens)

The first mating season of queens takes place when they are between five and eight months old. However, they should not be allowed to mate until they are at least nine months old. The gestation period is sixty-three days. Tom cats usually begin mating at six to eight months of age.

The best age to have a cat desexed is between four and five months old for females and at about six months for males.

Queens have two or three breeding seasons a year and three to four heats during these seasons. A queen can, and if given the opportunity will, mate again when her kittens are about four weeks old.

Since the average queen can produce as many as three to four litters a year, the question of whether to have your queen spayed is of some relevance to conscientious cat owners.

---

97 Milk Fever (Eclampsia)

This condition may be seen in all queens, but it occurs more frequently in those which have just had large litters. It usually manifests itself just before the kittens are weaned – about five or six weeks after birth.

Cause
Calcium deficiency.

Symptoms
1 The queen becomes very restless. She miaows a great deal and lies with her legs extended, breathing rapidly.
2 She may lose her sense of co-ordination, and when she tries to stand, she falls over.
3 This stage is associated with a rise in temperature, up to 107°F (41°C).
4 Dribbling, rigidity and convulsions.

WARNING
Do not allow the queen's symptoms to progress so far. If she is in this state and left untreated, she will die.

Treatment
Treatment is simple, but it must be given by a vet. It consists of feeding calcium borogluconate intravenously. If convulsions have not started, owners can mix 4 oz (100 g) calcium borogluconate with 1 pint (500 ml) water, and give the solution by mouth until the symptoms stop, or the vet arrives.

Prevention
During lactation, give plenty of milk and bone-meal. Give half a teaspoon of bone-meal to the queen every day.

---

98 Mother Cat eating her Kittens

A queen having her first litter should be carefully watched, for in certain circumstances she may attempt to eat her young.

This is not as monstrous nor as abnormal as it sounds. It may be the result of a natural fright response, but more often it is caused by a faulty placenta-eating instinct. In this case, the mother simply does not know where the placenta (after-birth) ends and her new-born kittens begin.

---

99 Motion Sickness

This condition is common in cats.

Symptoms
Restlessness, excessive salivation and persistent vomiting.

Treatment
(i)   Before the trip, administer an animal tranquillizer (these can be obtained from a vet). It is never a good idea to give a cat a tranquillizer intended for human consumption, since there is a vast difference in correct dosage.
(ii)   However, in extraordinary circumstances, if animal tranquillizers are not available, preparations for human travel sickness, available from chemists, may have to be used instead. Kwells, Marzine or Dramine will serve. An oral dose of 2 mg per 1 lb ($\frac{1}{2}$ kg) body weight should not be exceeded. The exact dosage will depend on the size of the animal.

Prevention
(i)   Before long journeys, withhold all food for twelve hours. But give your cat plenty of water.
(ii)   An effective way of preventing car sickness is to get your cat accustomed to car travel by taking it on short trips when possible. Also, allow the cat to spend time in the car when it is not in use.

100 Nasal Discharge

See also **Sinusitis.**

A thick yellowy mucus may suggest one of the feline virus diseases. Normally, a healthy cat's nose is cold and wet. A hot dry nose suggests a fever, illness, and warrants further investigation. Obviously, a vet must be consulted.

101 Neuralgia

Cause
Nerve pain.

Symptoms
1 Sudden and obvious pain.
2 The muscles of the cat's neck, back, or legs, depending upon where the neuralgia is being experienced, grow very tense.
3 These attacks of neuralgia are intermittent, and may last for several hours.

Treatment
(i) Keep the cat warm and allow it to rest.
(ii) An infra-red lamp is a great comfort to a cat suffering from neuralgia. Mount the lamp about three feet over the cat's bed and leave it on all night. In the absence of an infra-red lamp, an electric blanket or hot water bottle is also helpful.
(iii) Administer half of a 300 mg Paracetamol tablet. Do not repeat dosage for 72 hours. See **Tablets and Pills: Techniques of Administration.**

102 Nipple Soreness

See also **Inability to give Milk.**

Cause
This condition is seen fairly often while the female is nursing litter. It is caused by the nails of the kittens pricking the soft flesh of the teats.

Symptoms
1   The kittens will be screaming for food.
2   The queen's nipples will be red and cracked.

Treatment
(i)   If the nipples are simply sore and red, apply lanolin or vaseline twice a day. If vaseline is used, make certain that it is rubbed in well. Wipe off any surplus vaseline with cotton wool.
(ii)   If the nipples have become cracked, bathe them three times a day in a solution made from ½ teaspoon (2½ ml) boracic acid added to ½ pint (250 ml) water. After bathing, dry the nipples gently but thoroughly with cotton wool and apply lanolin or vaseline.

Prevention
The nails of kittens should not be clipped or cut. They should be filed once a week (see illustration 10).

Filing a Kitten's Nails   10

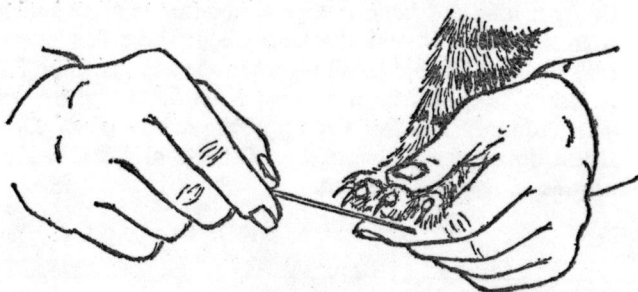

103 Nosebleed (Epistaxis)

Nosebleeds are symptoms, and the cat owner should be more concerned with the cause than with the nosebleed itself. In most instances a nosebleed will stop of its own accord fairly quickly.

Causes
Nosebleeds can be the result of:
1 Car accidents.
2 Tumours.
3 Decayed tooth sockets.
4 Excessive sneezing.
5 Foreign bodies in the nose.
6 High blood pressure.
7 Minute parasites in the nose.

Treatment
(i) The nostrils should be sponged dry with cotton wool.
(ii) Get a good light and carefully examine the nostrils to see if the cause or site of the haemorrhage is visible. If you can see a foreign body, you may remove it with tweezers. If you cannot see anything, do not poke about in the cat's nostrils. The mucous membrane, which lines the nostrils, is very sensitive and easily injured.
(iii) If the cause of the nosebleed is not visible, then keep the cat as still as possible. Apply cold compresses or ice cubes to the bridge of the nose.
(iv) If this treatment does not stop the bleeding, or if the bleeding continues intermittently, get professional assistance. The degree of urgency can be determined by the severity of the bleeding.

Tip of the nose
Bleeding from the tip of the nose can be both persistent and, if too much blood is lost, potentially dangerous. It can be controlled by pressure with the fingers

104 Nursing

If your pet is suffering from a severe or debilitating disease, and is too weak and sick to groom and feed itself, the nursing and loving care it receives from you will have a vital effect upon its recovery. This care extends to grooming and hygiene as well as to proper feeding.

(i)   Keep sick cats in a warm, quiet dimly lit place. Try not to disturb them.

(ii)   Keep sick cats clean. Special care should be taken if they are suffering from diarrhoea or vomiting, for psychological as well as sanitary reasons. All cats are fastidious and become distressed if allowed to foul themselves. If this occurs they should be gently washed with soap and water. A little talcum powder dusted on after washing is helpful.

(iii)   Apart from doing what is necessary for their well-being, leave sick cats alone as much as possible. There is a difference between loving care and fussing. Do not fuss over a sick cat.

Diet

Sick cats and cats recuperating from an illness need nourishing food even if they do not always want it. Supplement their diet with a mixture of 4 tablespoons glucose powder to 1 pint (500 ml) water daily, to supply extra energy. Serve this mixture in place of the cat's regular drinking water. Do not give this or any fluids to a cat which is vomiting. See **Excessive Drinking**. If the cat does have an appetite, do not give it all it wants at one time. Rather, feed it small amounts at frequent intervals.

If the cat has no appetite, try to tempt it with strong-smelling foods such as kippers, cheese, chicken, chicken livers, fish, smoked salmon or tinned sardines. A cat's sense of smell, if properly enticed, will often start it eating again. If none of these work, try making a home-made meat extract. This is made by mincing raw meat as fine as possible and pouring the boiling water over the minced meat. The resulting liquid is then poured into a bowl and a pinch of salt and a tiny pinch of monosodium glutamate are added to bring out the flavour.

Make every effort to tempt the cat to eat voluntarily. If nothing works, you will have to force-feed. This is a last resort. Remember, the smallest amount of food taken voluntarily will do more good than a much larger amount which has been force-fed. See **Force-Feeding**.

Hygiene

All bowls, dishes, spoons, etc , which come into contact with the cat must be sterilized in boiling water after each meal. Scrupulous hygiene is absolutely essential to successful nursing.

Nursing diabetic cats
See also **Diabetes.**
The diabetic cat requires a diet high in protein and low in carbohydrates. Fortunately, most tinned animal foods are of this composition and provide adequate nourishment when supplemented with two raw eggs per week, mixed into the cat's food to supply the necessary amount of fat. Diabetic cats should not be fed dry animal foods.

Nursing elderly cats
Elderly cats present special problems, and their general condition can be greatly improved by feeding good-quality foods in proper amounts. See **Diet.**

When nursing an older cat whose appetite is sluggish, stimulate the appetite by feeding meat extracts and flavourings. Since a cat's sense of smell and taste diminish with age, some extra attention to diet is necessary to keep the sick elderly cat eating. Remember, cats will not eat food that they cannot smell.

Most elderly cats are nephritic, that is, they suffer from kidney problems and should be fed a low-protein diet, composed of white meat (rabbit, fish or chicken) with carbohydrates, in the form of rice or biscuit meal, mixed into their food. A few cats hate rice and biscuit meal. Faced with this problem, the best solution is to put the rice or biscuit meal into a blender and then mix it very well with some food that the animal does like. If necessary, special therapeutic diets are available from a vet. Supplement the cat's diet with Vitamin A and Vitamin B12, contained in Abidec drops and Cytacon tablets respectively. These are available from chemists. See **Tablets and Pills: Techniques of Administration.**

Elderly cats should be given all the water they require. Make sure that the cat's drinking bowl is always full.

Nursing young cats
Diet is of importance in the successful nursing of young cats. When cats develop infections, their food intake falls. This is particularly dangerous with kittens, which are very dependent upon daily nutrition. When they stop eating, they begin a cycle of malnutrition and further infection, ultimately ending in death.

A young cat weighing 2 lb (1 kg) requires at least 8 teaspoons (40 ml) water daily. It also needs minerals, proteins, carbohydrates, fats and vitamins. See **Diet.**

As long as there is no diarrhoea or vomiting, add powdered cow's milk, at twice the strength recommended for human babies, to the kitten's diet.

For orphan kittens, milk substitutes such as Lactol or Welpi may be given. Feed every two hours for the first week, day and night. Afterwards, every three hours for ten days.

If there is diarrhoea or vomiting, then neither milk nor milk products should be given. With diarrhoea or vomiting, withhold all food for twelve hours, then give a mixture of ½ pint (250 ml) water, 3 tablespoons glucose powder, 1 raw egg white and 1 pinch salt. Small portions of boned chicken or rice may be given three or four times a day for four days.

If, after twenty-four hours, the kitten still refuses to eat, a vet should be consulted. If a vet is not available, force-feed it with Brands Essence until food is taken voluntarily. Continue the water and glucose mixture as well, force-feeding if necessary.

---

105 Opening a Cat's Mouth

Technique
To put it mildly, cats can be very difficult about having their mouths opened, but if it must be done, there are two ways of doing it.

With assistant
Ideally, you should have an assistant. The assistant holds the cat while you approach from behind. Then (assuming you are right-handed) place your left hand on top of the cat's head, and the thumb and index finger behind the upper canines (fangs), a finger on each side. Place the remaining fingers of the left hand behind the animal's ears and pivot its head backwards. At the same time open its jaw with your right hand.

Without assistant
If no assistant is available and you have to do the job yourself, wrap the cat in a large, thick towel, so that only its head protrudes. Then place your thumb and index finger behind the upper canines, the remaining fingers behind the cat's ears. Pivot the head backwards, and at the same time apply slight pressure with your thumb and index finger. This will force the cat to open its mouth.

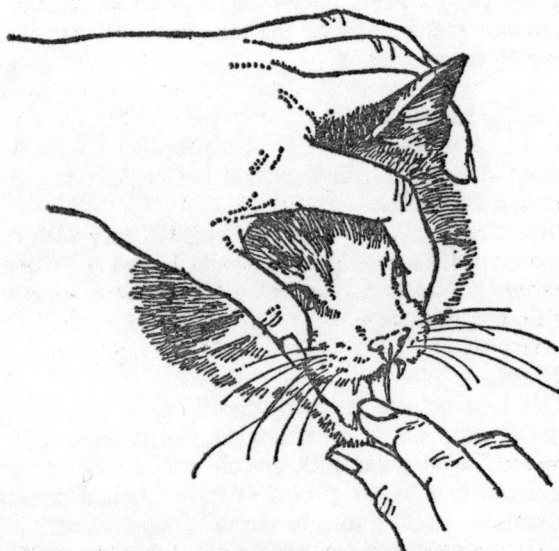

The procedure should be carried out in a calm but determined manner. The secret is to know exactly what you are going to do before you start to do it.

---

106 Orphan Kittens

Very young kittens (up to four weeks old) without a mother, or those from a mother unable to feed them (see **Inability to give Milk**), should be placed in a small warm box and fed on a substitute milk supplement, such as Lactol or Welpi, every two hours day and night for the first two weeks. After that they should be fed every three hours.

After each feeding they should be burped: rub the abdomen gently with an oiled finger so you do not irritate the kitten's tender skin. This burping is normally accompanied by urination and defecation.

Homemade milk supplement

If commercial substitutes are not available, you can make your own milk supplement, composed of 30 oz (900 ml) cow's milk, 1 egg yolk, 1 pinch bone-meal, 1 pinch citric acid. Stir the mixture and keep it in the refrigerator. Warm it to 100°F (37°C) before feeding.

Feeding technique

(i) Use an eyedropper or doll's feeding bottle. Be sure to clean thoroughly and then boil the dropper or doll's bottle after each feeding.

(ii) The amount of food required will vary with the size of the animal. Generally, they should be fed according to their appetite. Unfortunately, some kittens have appetites larger than their capacity.

Diarrhoea

Overfeeding may result in diarrhoea. Should diarrhoea develop, withhold the milk supplement and give the kitten luke-warm boiled water with glucose added. (Three tablespoons glucose powder to 1 pint (500 ml) boiled water). If the diarrhoea stops, return to the milk supplement.

If the diarrhoea persists for more than twenty-four hours, call a vet. If the diarrhoea was not caused by overfeeding, it may be the result of an infection.

Solid Food

After three weeks, kittens will show an interest in more adult food. Encourage this new appetite by feeding them bits of boned chicken, fish and minced meat. If these delicacies are not available, tinned or dry cat foods may be given in their place.

Weaning

Weaning, which means taking young animals off their mother's milk, or off the milk supplement, should be completed by the time the kitten is four to six weeks old.

---

107   Pain

Symptoms

There is no register for pain. The cat owner must observe his pet's reactions as a guide to the location and severity of the pain. Cats show pain by assuming an abnormal position, or by abnormal behaviour.

Pain in different parts of the body produces different reactions. For example:

Pain in the legs produces lameness.

Pain in the abdomen causes restlessness, sitting or lying in abnormal positions, and whining. There is also a tendency to seek out cold places, such as cement floors, to lie on.

Pain in the head produces languor. The cat paws at its head, is restless, and may press its head against the wall.

Acute pain causes the cat to cry, whine, whimper and act frightened. It will look at, or lick, the affected area.

A cat manifesting symptoms of pain should be carefully observed. Its behaviour may give you a clue to the problem. For example, a cat with a foreign body in its paw will chew at its foot, while a cat with a foreign body in its mouth will paw at its mouth.

---

108 Paint, Removal of

Technique

(i) Get some dry cloths and rub off all the paint you can.

(ii) Then wash small areas thoroughly with soap and water and keep rubbing with dry cloths.

(iii) Snip off patches of matted hair with scissors.

(iv) For particularly difficult patches, pour a little gin or rubbing alcohol on to the patch and then rub it off with a dry cloth. Hand cleaners, such as Swarfega, may be used.

WARNING

Never use paraffin, kerosene, turpentine or any of the paint solvents. They cause burns on the cat's skin.

Lead in paints

Paints which contain lead are poisonous when ingested. If a cat has eaten paint with a lead base, or has licked lead paint off its coat, force-feed a bowl of milk with the whites of two eggs beaten into it. See **Force-Feeding**.

If lead poisoning is suspected, do not try to induce vomiting.

If the cat is in pain, or is covered in paint, get it to a vet. A cat with paint on its fur will try to lick the paint off, and though it probably won't succeed in getting all the paint off, it will probably succeed in licking off enough to poison itself. See **Poisoning**.

Often, a cat covered in paint requires a general anaesthetic so that the fur can be combed out or clipped.

In severe cases, the pain caused by the paint on the skin can drive the animal into a state of shock, requiring intravenous fluids and other professional treatment.

109　Pleurisy

Pleurisy refers to a specific inflammation of the pleura, the membrane which surrounds the lungs and lines the walls of the chest.

Symptoms
Pleurisy produces the same symptoms as pneumonia; a high temperature, painful and difficult breathing, loss of appetite, and lethargy.

Treatment
(i)　Pleurisy, like pneumonia, cannot be accurately diagnosed nor adequately treated by the non-professional.

(ii)　Home treatment consists of keeping the cat warm, and trying to get it to take nourishment and to drink plenty of fluids.

(iii)　It must be stressed that pleurisy should be considered a serious illness. Suspicion of pleurisy warrants an immediate consultation with a vet.

110　Pneumonia

Pneumonia is an infection of the lungs, quite common in cats.

Causes
This lung infection can be caused by viruses, bacteria, or worms. Sometimes, a simple chill or cold, if left untreated, can develop into pneumonia.

Symptoms
1　General symptoms include: coughing, lethargy and dullness, high body temperature.

2　Also check the cat for bluish tinges of the mucous membranes.

3 There may be a definite rattling and bubbling in the cat's chest.

4 Often the afflicted cat will lie on its breastbone, with its elbows stuck out at an angle of forty-five degrees. This is caused by the sore chest that accompanies pneumonia.

5 When the cat is picked up, there is further evidence of pain in its chest, because its lungs are sore and picking it up compresses the lungs and increases the soreness.

Treatment

(i) Pneumonia must be considered a serious disease, and professional assistance is necessary.

(ii) If a vet is not immediately available, the cat owner must make certain that the animal is kept warm. Wrap it in a blanket or a woolly sweater, or button a cardigan round it.

(iii) Also, be sure that the room where the cat is kept is warm; at the same time, make sure that there is adequate fresh air.

(iv) Try to tempt the cat's appetite with light nourishing foods.

(v) Give plenty of fluids.

III Poisoning

Before proceeding to more detailed information regarding symptoms and treatments for common poisons, it is essential to realize that in most cases it is just not possible for the cat owner to diagnose accurately a specific case of poisoning from observation of symptoms alone. The only exception is when the owner has actually seen his cat eating a particular poison.

In the majority of instances, treatment must be general.

Symptoms

These are so broad as to include vomiting, diarrhoea, internal haemorrhage, inco-ordination, twitching, convulsions, coma and unconsciousness.

A glance at this list makes it obvious that all these symptoms are also present in many other conditions. Without further evidence, it is difficult to be certain that they are caused by poison.

However, if there are reasonable grounds to suspect that an animal has eaten poison, and providing the cat is conscious, the first rule is to make it vomit as soon as possible.

Technique for inducing vomiting
The simplest and fastest way to induce vomiting in an animal is to throw ordinary table salt into the back of its mouth: 1 teaspoon (5 ml) salt is sufficient. See **Opening a Cat's Mouth.**

WARNING
The exception to this rule is when acid, lead or other corrosive poisons have been ingested, in which case vomiting is not desirable. When acid or corrosive poisons are suspected, give olive oil, by mouth, up to $\frac{1}{4}$ pint (125 ml).

Subsequent treatment
Subsequent treatment consists of administering the proper antidote (providing you can identify the poison) and treating any symptoms as they arise.

Otherwise, administer the universal antidote (see below).

Universal antidote
When the type of poison is unknown, administer what is hopefully known as a universal antidote, consisting of:
  2 parts charcoal (burnt toast)
  1 part magnesium oxide (milk of magnesia)
  1 part tannic acid (strong tea)
Give 2 teaspoons (5 ml) of the above mixture. See **Force-Feeding.**

General Note
If possible, always bring a sample of the suspected poison and a sample of the cat's vomit to the vet, along with the patient. If the poison can be quickly determined, much valuable time can be saved.

If the cat is unconscious
(i) Get the cat to a vet. Do not induce vomiting.
(ii) Make sure the tongue is out. Prop open the jaw with a cotton reel.

If the cat was in physical contact with toxic or corrosive substances
Wash the affected area with liberal amounts of clean water. Do not use soap.

If the animal has been in physical contact with a non-corrosive substance
If a non-corrosive poison has contacted the skin or fur, bathe the affected portions with soap and water. Even if the poison does not burn the skin, it must be removed immediately; otherwise, the cat will lick its fur and ingest the poison.

If the animal is hyperexcited or having convulsions
Protect the cat from hurting itself by following the procedure for fits and convulsions. See **Fits (Convulsions)**.

Acid poisoning
Common acid poisons
Sulphuric acid (found in defoliants and car batteries), nitric acid, hydrochloric acid, spirits of salt.

Symptoms
1 Inflamed patches on skin, which when licked cause:
2 Burning of the mouth.
3 Profuse dribbling.
4 Vomiting.

Treatment
(i) Administer 4 tablespoons (100 ml) of a solution made by adding 2 tablespoons sodium bicarbonate to 1 pint (500 ml) water.
(ii) Force-feed 4 tablespoons (100 ml) of a solution made by adding 1 egg white to ½ pint (250 ml) milk. See **Force-Feeding**.
(iii) For acid burns, apply bicarbonate of soda to the affected areas of the skin. Make a solution by adding 2 tablespoons bicarbonate to 1 pint (500 ml) water.
(iv) Seek professional help.

Alkali poisoning
Common alkali poisons
Caustic soda, caustic potash.

Symptoms
Soapy patches on the fur, dribbling, etc.

Treatment
(i) Administer 2 tablespoons (50 ml) of a mixture made by adding 1/10 pint (50 ml) vinegar to 1 pint (500 ml) water.
(ii) Wash the mouth out with vinegar.

(iii) For alkali burns, apply vinegar by pouring it directly over the burn, or by saturating a rag with vinegar and applying the rag to the burn.
(iv) Get professional help.

WARNING
Do not induce vomiting.

Arsenic poisoning
Sources
Rat and mouse poisons; ant poisons; insecticides; sheep and cattle dips; around smelting works and mines. Arsenic is also a common impurity found in many chemicals.

Symptoms
Acute arsenic poisoning may lead to death so quickly that there is no time to observe symptoms.

Smaller doses of arsenic produce symptoms which include intense abdominal pain, vomiting, staggering, diarrhoea, collapse, coma, and finally, death.

The breath of a cat suffering from arsenic poisoning will have a strong smell of garlic.

Treatment
If the cat is conscious:
(i) Induce vomiting by giving 2 teaspoons (10 ml) salt, by mouth.
(ii) Force-feed the cat 4 tablespoons (100 ml) of a solution made by adding 2 tablespoons bicarbonate of soda to 1 pint (500 ml) water.
(iii) Give the cat an enema of warm soapy water. See **Enema**.
(iv) Administer demulcents (substances which cover the irritated stomach lining), such as milk, glycerine and water, barley water, or starch and water mixed to a thin paste.

Benzoic acid poisoning
Benzoic acid is a preservative which is added to slab meat (processed meat) purchased from pet shops. Quite frequently, manufacturers add too much benzoic acid to their product, and the result is that they poison the pets they are supposed to be feeding.

Symptoms
1 The symptoms range from staggering and drowsiness to

severe hallucinations which produce markedly abnormal, overexcited behaviour. This is the classic cat-on-a-hot-tin-roof symptom.

2 Very severe cases of benzoic acid poisoning can result in sudden death.

Treatment
(i) Confine your cat. Put it in a quiet, dark room and contact the vet. The effects of benzoic acid poisoning usually wear off after two or three days.
(ii) Give no food or water for twenty-four hours.
(iii) Do not attempt to induce vomiting.

Insulin poisoning
Usually occurs within an hour after insulin treatment.

Cause
Diabetic cats receiving insulin treatment at home may be inadvertantly overdosed.

Symptoms
These vary from staggering and inco-ordination to unconsciousness.

Treatment
(i) If the cat is still conscious, give it 5 lumps of sugar. Break the lumps into tablet-sized pieces to make it easier to administer, and easier for the cat to swallow. See **Tablets and Pills: Techniques of Administration.** If only powdered sugar is available, calculate one lump of sugar equals ½ teaspoon of powdered sugar.
(ii) If the cat has lost consciousness and a vet is not immediately available, mix the sugar with water. Crush the sugar lumps between spoons to make the sugar dissolve faster, and pour a little at a time into the cat's mouth.

Mercury poisoning
Sources
Antiseptics and fungicides, broken thermometers and barometers, ointments containing mercury.

Symptoms
Early symptoms are vomiting and diarrhoea.
  If death does not occur immediately from shock, the early

symptoms are followed by ulceration of the mouth and tongue and acute kidney failure.

Treatment
The absorption of mercury into the system is very rapid, and swift treatment is essential.

If the cat's stomach can be emptied within half an hour of ingestion, then there is a good chance of recovery.
(i)   Induce vomiting.
(ii) The cat should then be force-fed raw egg whites and milk. See **Force-Feeding**.
(iii) Induce vomiting again.

Phosphorus poisoning
Sources
Red-tipped matches; rat and mouse poisons; cockroach poisons; the striking surfaces of matchboxes; fireworks.

Symptoms
1   The classic symptoms of staggering, abdominal pain and vomiting are present. But if phosphorus poisoning is suspected, pay particular attention to the vomit, which will glow in the dark. The cat's breath and vomit will have a strong smell of garlic.
2   Following the onset of these symptoms, there is a period of apparent recovery, which may last from three to four hours to several days.
3   This recovery period then ends, and the abdominal pain and vomiting recur, together with jaundice – a yellowish tinge appearing in the eyes and the mucous membranes – and nervous symptoms which, if ignored, will lead to coma and death.

Treatment
Treatment must not be delayed.
(i)   At the first suspicion of phosphorus poisoning, induce vomiting.
(ii) After causing the cat to vomit, force-feed it a solution of 1 teaspoon (5 ml) 1 per cent copper sulphate to 1 pint water.
(iii) Induce vomiting again.
(iv) Administer 1 teaspoon potassium permanganate in 1 pint (500 ml) water.
(v)   Give the cat an enema of warm soapy water. See **Enema**.
(vi) Do not give any fats, even milk, for the next five days.

Strychnine poisoning
Sources
Rat and mouse and mole poisons.

Symptoms
The first symptoms of strychnine poisoning are excessive nervousness, restlessness, noticeable twitching of the muscles, and stiffness of the neck.

As the condition progresses, these symptoms become more pronounced and convulsions suddenly occur.

In convulsions caused by strychnine poisoning, the limbs are extended and the neck is curved upwards and backwards.

During the early stages, these convulsions are sporadic, but they will become progressively more frequent, until any external stimulus – the slightest noise of touch, even a current of air – will produce them.

During the latter stage, the iris is widely dilated, covering nearly the whole surface of the eyeball.

Finally, death is caused by the inability to breathe, due to paralysis of the respiratory muscles.

Treatment
(i)   If the cat is having convulsions, the best treatment is to have the cat anaesthetized by a vet. Do not try to take the cat to the vet; you will not make it. Have the vet come to the cat.
(ii)   It is extremely difficult to move a convulsing cat. If you attempt to confine it in a closed basket, the cat runs the risk of choking on its own vomit. But if there is no other way, and you must transport the cat, try to glance inside the box or basket from time to time to make sure this has not happened.
(iii)   If a vet can be reached by telephone and if convulsions have not yet begun, get someone to contact a vet while you induce vomiting.
(iv)   After vomiting, force-feed the cat strong, cold tea. See **Force-Feeding.**
(v)   Further treatment must be left to a vet.
(vi)   While waiting for the vet, keep the cat very quiet and insulated from any external stimuli which might trigger off the convulsions. Place the cat in a quiet, darkened room.

Vomiting induced by poisons
The group of poisons which cause vomiting includes most of the common poisons such as arsenic, phosphorus and decayed foods.

Symptoms
1 Burns in the cat's mouth or on its tongue.
2 The vomit will give off a pronounced acid smell.

Treatment
Administer 2 tablespoons (50 ml) corn oil to soothe the stomach lining. Alternatively, use 3 tablespoons sodium bicarbonate to ½ pint (250 ml) water. See **Force-Feeding**.

WARNING
Do not administer emetics to animals which are already vomiting.

---

112   Post-Puerperal Metritis

This is an infection of the womb, producing an abnormal vaginal discharge that occurs shortly after the queen has given birth.

Symptoms
1 Symptoms of this condition appear in the mother two to five days after she has had her litter.
2 There is a heavy, dark, bloody discharge from the vagina. This should not be confused with the slight, greenish-brown discharge which is normal after a cat has had a litter.
3 Increased thirst.
4 High temperature. The normal discharge is not accompanied by high temperature and greatly increased thirst.

Treatment
Treatment must be given by a vet. The above symptoms merit his immediate attention.

---

113   Poultices

Use
The application of heat to a swelling or to a sore area will relieve the pain and control the swelling.

The advantage of a poultice is that it retains its heat without having to be constantly changed. There are several types of poultice, but the simplest, and one of the most effective, is a kaolin poultice. (Kaolin is available in tins, from all chemists.)

The poultice is prepared by heating the tin in a saucepanful of boiling water. When the clay is fairly hot, it is spread on a bandage, which is then taped over the affected area.

Before placing the bandage on the cat, test a bit of the kaolin on the back of your hand. It should be very warm, but not hot enough to cause you any pain.

The poultice should be changed every four hours.

Substitutes

If kaolin is not available, a poultice may be made from bread or from potatoes.

To make a poultice from bread, boil some water, soak a piece of bread in the boiling water, allow it to cool enough for you to handle it, then apply it to a bandage and tape the bandage to the affected area.

To make a poultice from potatoes, simply mash some freshly cooked potatoes, apply them to a bandage and tape the bandage over the affected area.

---

114 Prolapse of the Rectum

One of those conditions which look much worse than they really are. Actually it is fairly common in kittens suffering from persistent diarrhoea. Occasionally it is seen in older cats as well.

Treatment
(i)   Wash your hands.
(ii) Gently wash the area around the anus with warm soapy water.
(iii) Apply liquid paraffin liberally around the anal area.
(iv) Gently push back the protruding portion until the anus is normal.
(v)   Wash your hands again.
(vi) Contact the vet.

---

115 Prolapsed Third Eyelid

This condition, seen in cats, indicates a mild illness, such as slight nephritis, or a mild case of cat flu.

E

Description
The third eyelid comes from the inner corner of the eye and covers the entire eyeball. When this third eyelid is prolapsed, it does not retract normally, but remains covering part or all of the eyeball.

Treatment
(i) There is no need to treat the prolapsed eyelid, since it is only a symptom of other more generalized conditions. Give the cat extra vitamins: One 50 mg tablet of Vitamin B12 twice a day, plus one capsule of Vitamin A 500 international units per day. Be careful not to exceed the recommended vitamin dosage. See **Tablets and Pills: Techniques of Administration.**

(ii) If the cat is eating normally, there is no cause for alarm. But if the third eyelid does not return to normal within three to four days, have the cat looked at by a vet.

---

116   Pulse Taking

Place your index and middle finger over the femoral artery at the point where it crosses the thigh bone on the inside of the thigh, almost in the groin.

Count the pulse beats for ten seconds and multiply by six.

The pulse rate varies from one hundred and ten to one hundred and forty beats a minute when the cat is in good health.

A very slow pulse, thirty to fifty beats a minute, implies that the cat is very ill and requires immediate professional treatment. A very low pulse rate appears in cases of sedative overdose and in the final, declining stages of infection.

With a cat running a fever, there will be a persistent high pulse rate, which may be as fast as one hundred and sixty beats a minute. This also demands immediate professional treatment.

It is important for the cat owner to know his own pet's normal pulse rate when the animal is in good health, so that a higher or lower pulse rate will not go unnoticed.

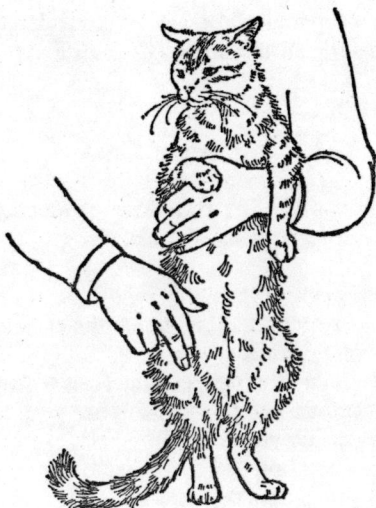

___

117 Pyometra

This condition is usually seen in older (five to six years old) females.

Cause
A pus-producing, abnormal development of the cells lining the womb. The condition occurs in two forms.

Symptoms
1 In the open form, there is a creamy, foul-smelling, vaginal discharge. Along with the discharge the queen will develop an increased thirst. There will also be some degree of abdominal enlargement. This is often confused with pregnancy.
However, pyometra is not an infectious disease, so there will not be any dramatic rise in body temperature.
2 In the closed form, there is no visible sign of discharge. The reason is that in this form the queen's cervix remains closed, and the uterus gradually fills up with pus.
This produces a pronounced enlargement of the abdomen, extreme lethargy and increased thirst.

Treatment
Both forms of pyometra must be considered serious, and they require surgical treatment. Consult a vet immediately.

---

118   Restraint: The Handling of Cats

By restraint we mean the technique of *handling, moving* and *holding* a cat largely against its will.

When to use restraint
When one must do something which the cat finds frightening, painful or objectionable.

It is never pleasant to use restraint, but when it is necessary, be firm and unhurried and know what you are going to do *before* you approach your cat.

There are several methods of restraining reluctant animals. The method you choose depends upon the temperament of the cat, and upon your purpose in restraining the cat. Do you want to move the animal or to hold it?

Technique
(i)   Difficult cats may be captured by throwing a coat or blanket over them and handling them through it.
(ii)   Quieter cats may be scruffed. To hold a cat by its scruff, take a firm grip, from behind, on the loose flesh just behind the animal's head. Hold tightly enough to prevent the cat from turning its head, but not so tightly that you cause it pain.
(iii)   Wrap the cat in a blanket, with its head showing.

---

119   Rickets

Causes
Rickets are the result of a calcium, phosphorus and Vitamin D deficiency.

Symptoms
Rickets affect young cats from three weeks to six months old. The first sign is usually a noticeable swelling of the wrist joint. Swellings will also be observed along the side of the chest. Severe cases will eventually develop bending of the long leg bones, causing bow-leggedness.

Treatment
(i) Mix sterilized bone-flour into the cat's food. (Half teaspoon daily).
(ii) Give Abidec drops (two to three drops daily).
(iii) Administration of cod liver oil is not recommended for young cats suffering from rickets, since cod liver oil can remove the calcium from the bones if given in excess of two to three drops daily.
(iv) Seek professional help.

120 Ringworm

Ringworm is a disease of the top layer of the skin (the epidermis) caused by two groups of fungi, *both of which are contagious and can affect human beings.*

Symptoms
Ringworm is fairly common in cats. Breaks in the skin, which take the form of dry scaly patches, circular in shape, are found on the head and chest and paws. These lesions are accompanied by a collection of grey flakes in the fur, like cigarette ash. This stage is followed by the characteristic circular patches described above.

Treatment
Always wash your hands after treating a cat suffering from ringworm.
(i) Clip the hair around the breaks in the skin.
(ii) Apply a dilute solution of Cetavlon to the lesions and the surrounding area: 1 teaspoon (5 ml) Cetavlon to 10 teaspoons (50 ml) water. Saturate cotton wool in the solutions and continue the applications for as long as the breaks in the skin are visible.
(iii) The specific and most successful treatment for ringworm is the oral administration of griseofulvin tablets, available from vets or doctors.

In healthy cats, the condition may disappear spontaneously in about two months. But do not wait two months, because in addition to being contagious to people, ringworm is a highly unpleasant and very uncomfortable disease and should be treated on first sight.

---

121   **Saline Solution**

Literally, a sterile (germ-free) salt solution.
(i)   Dissolve 1 teaspoon block or cooking salt (iodine-free salt) in 1 pint (500 ml) boiling water.
(ii) Allow the water to cool to body temperature, then apply.

---

122   **Sedative Overdose**

Sedatives, in the form of sleeping pills, are often left around by careless owners and eaten by unwary pets.

Symptoms
1   The cat will stagger about and appear very drowsy. It will keep trying to go to sleep.
2   There may or may not be an empty pill container to confirm your suspicions. The animal may have eaten the container along with the pills.

Treatment
(i)   Contact a vet immediately.
(ii) Induce vomiting.
(iii) Administer stimulants. Strong tea or black coffee, cooled, should also be given.
(iv) Keep the animal awake, until the effects wear off.
   If the cat keeps falling asleep, slap its face to keep it awake.

---

123   **Shampooing a Cat**

The amount of difficulty experienced in shampooing a cat depends primarily upon the cat. Some cats will co-operate, others will not. A cat which is accustomed to being handled and groomed is more likely to permit a shampoo without too much fuss.
   Difficult cats require an assistant. Have the assistant scruff the cat while you do the shampooing. See **Restraint.** Be careful not to get soap into the animal's eyes, or it will be twice as difficult next time you shampoo the cat.
   If there is no one to help you, put the cat into a pillowcase with just its head protruding, and shampoo it through the pillowcase.

124 Shock

Shock is the term used to describe a state which is characterized by an acute and progressive failure of the circulatory system.

Causes
While the exact causes of shock are unknown, the condition follows most forms of severe injury, massive haemorrhages, heart failure, serious burns, anaemia and dehydration.

Symptoms
(Following severe trauma, i.e. serious accidents): apathy; low body temperature; pale gums and pale tongue; a rapid thready pulse; rapid shallow breathing; thirst; and finally, complete collapse.

Treatment
(i) First aid treatment consists of keeping the cat warm by wrapping it in a blanket. Keep the cat as quiet as possible and get it to a vet.
(ii) The prime form of treatment is to restore the amount of circulating fluid in the blood vessels through a transfusion, which can be administered by the vet.

125 Sinusitis

Sinusitis is an infection of the sinuses. (The sinuses are an extension of the nasal chamber, located in the front of the head.)

Causes
The infection may be caused either by germs or by a foreign body in the nose.

Symptoms
Except in the case of foreign bodies, sinusitis rarely occurs on its own. It is usually seen as a sequel to virus conditions, such as cat flu.
   The symptoms themselves are:
1 A yellowish nasal discharge.
2 Bouts of sneezing.
3 Loss of appetite.

Treatment

Since many other illnesses are characterized by these same symptoms, you will need professional help to make a definite diagnosis. So, if the symptoms continue for more than twenty-four hours, take the cat to a vet. (If it is sinusitis, he will probably administer a course of antibiotics.)

If a vet is not immediately available, home treatment consists of

(i) keeping the cat's face clean of the mucous discharge, and
(ii) assisting the cat to breathe normally by clearing the nasal passages.

This is accomplished by inhalations of a preparation of Friars Balsam or menthol in hot water. To make this preparation, place some boiling water in a large, shallow, tin dish (e.g. a pie tin) and add 3 tablespoons of Friars Balsam or menthol to the boiling water. Then, calmly but firmly, hold the cat's face over the steam for a moment or two.

Try to treat this inhalation as an ordinary occurrence. The trick is to have the cat inhale as much of the vapour as possible; and this is only achieved if the cat is not alarmed.

Also, you do not want to hold a struggling frightened cat over boiling water, so do not force your cat, just handle it with confidence.

---

126 Skin Diseases: General

Cats can develop acute skin conditions very quickly. These conditions are very painful and very unhealthy and should not be allowed to continue. Prompt treatment by the cat owner can prevent nuisances from becoming serious problems.

The most obvious indication of skin problems is excessive scratching. Any cat that is continually scratching itself either has trouble or is heading for trouble. The owner must take note of this and set about discovering the cause.

Also, skin diseases have a public health aspect. Some, such as ringworm and sarcoptic mange, can be transmitted from animals to people. Many others are transmitted from animal to animal, e.g. demodectic mange.

Skin diseases take various forms and many factors are involved, but for purposes of home treatment, we can divide skin diseases into:

1 contagious (which means that they are transmitted by direct contact).

2 infectious (which means that they can be transmitted through the air), such as ringworm.

3 non-infectious and non-contagious, such as eczema, and diseases caused by hormonal imbalance.

Contagious

Contagious diseases, as well as fleas, lice, mange, mites, infectious ringworm, should be treated under strict hygienic conditions, and the affected cat should be kept away from other animals, and from small children.

Non-contagious

With non-contagious skin diseases, the owner may feel there is not the same urgency for treatment. Some owners, in time, even get used to their cat's condition and 'learn to live with it'. These owners would do better to learn to cure it.

Aside from the eventual worsening of the original complaint, neglect invites a host of secondary complications.

All abnormal skin conditions should be diagnosed and treated at once.

Hormonal imbalance

This is a common cause of non-contagious skin disease. The imbalance can produce bald spots as well as certain varieties of eczema in the cat. If the symptoms are observed and treatment is instituted early on, the condition can be quickly corrected.

Hereditary diseases

Owners of highly bred cats, especially those bred for certain abnormal traits, such as the squashed-nosed Persian, should be aware of the particular skin diseases their animal's breeding makes it heir to.

External origins

Chemicals, foreign bodies (such as grass seeds), even overexposure to light, can cause a skin disease.

Allergies

Probably the most common of non-contagious skin diseases are those caused by allergies. Unfortunately, they are also the most difficult to cure.

127 Slipped Disc

This condition is fairly rare among cats.

Causes
Accidents, obesity.

Symptoms
1 Acute pain when the cat attempts to walk.
2 In some cases, the cat cannot move its back legs.
3 There may be rigidity or tenseness of the abdomen. Touch the cat's stomach lightly. The skin may be as tight as a drum.
4 There may be retention of urine and faeces, at first. Then, as the bladder and the small intestine fill up, the cat is unable to control itself and there is involuntary passage of the body wastes.

Treatment
The first thing to do is to ease the cat's pain. See **Analgesics.** The severity of the symptoms indicates the severity of the condition, and while most mild instances of a slipped disc will right themselves, a vet should be consulted. If the condition persists or recurs frequently, surgery may be necessary.

128 Sneezing

Continual sneezing is a much more serious symptom in cats than in human beings.

Intermittent sneezing
If the cat sneezes on and off for a few hours, but otherwise seems all right – no temperature, apathy, etc – the cause of the sneezing is probably due to simple irritation, caused by a bit of dust up the nose.

Prolonged sneezing
If the cat continues to sneeze throughout the day, with accompanying nasal discharge, suspect an infection. Get professional assistance.

Bursts of strenuous sneezing
Strenuous and continued sneezing suggests a foreign body in the nose.

Examine the nostrils. You will need a good light for this. (An electric torch is ideal.) If the foreign object is visible, use tweezers to remove it carefully.

If you do not see anything, *do not poke about with your tweezers. The nasal lining is easily ruptured.* See **Nosebleed.**

---

129 Sprains and Strains

Sprains and strains are very similar in their effects and symptoms. A sprain involves the ligaments around a joint and a strain involves the muscles. In both cases the tissues are torn.

Causes
Sprains and strains are usually caused by violent exercise.

Symptoms
The diagnosis must often be made as the result of negative findings for fractures and dislocations and bites. After these have been eliminated as the cause of the cat's lameness, look for a slight swelling around the joint or muscle.

Treatment
(i)   Alternate hot and cold compresses over the swelling until it goes down.
(ii)   If the cat is very uncomfortable, administer analgesics.

---

130 Stains at the corner of the Eye

Certain cats, especially all-white cats, may develop brown staining in the corner of their eyes.

Cause
Blockage or absence of tear ducts.

Treatment
Make a very dilute solution of 20 vol hydrogen peroxide (1 part peroxide to 10 parts water) and bathe the stains liberally. *Do not bathe the eyeball, just the stains.*

131   Stings

Treatment

If you have seen the insect stinging your cat, try to locate the sting, which may be at the top of the swelling, and remove it by pinching at the bottom of the swelling with a pair of tweezers or a couple of wooden match sticks. Only bee stings stay in, because they are barbed.

Do not try to pull out the sting with your fingers. You will only succeed in making matters worse by squeezing the balance of the sting's contents into your cat.

Bee stings

Washing soda should be applied directly on to the bite. This will relieve the pain.

Wasp stings

For wasp stings, use vinegar. For bites in the mouth, use an ice pack to reduce the swelling.

EMERGENCY

Should the swelling – or, in the event of multiple bites, the swellings – become very large (golf-ball size or larger), or if the cat has difficulty in breathing, get the animal to a vet immediately. This is an emergency.

In these severe cases, if a vet is not available, try an animal-loving doctor, a dentist, even a pharmacist. An injection of antihistamine is necessary.

Mild cases

Fortunately, most stings are not so severe and the pain usually subsides in half an hour.

Treat mild discomfort in cats with half of a 500 mg Paracetamol tablet, once only. The cat's discomfort should not last longer than a day. If it does, professional assistance is needed.

132   Swallowing Safety Pins or other sharp Foreign Objects

Force-feed the cat bread or porridge. Also feed it small balls of cotton wool, which have been dipped in a meat extract, such as Bovril, for flavouring. See **Force-Feeding**.

Then obtain professional advice; an X-ray may be needed.

133 Swelling of the Abdomen

A sudden and dramatic increase in the size of the abdomen
suggests:
1 Overeating.
2 Pregnancy.
3 Tumours.
4 Fluid in the abdomen.
5 Pyometra.
6 Ovarian cyst.
7 Enlargement of the liver.
8 Enlargement of the spleen.

If the symptoms described under each of these subjects (see
Index) are similar to those exhibited by your cat, it is worth
paying a visit to your vet. When you first notice the signs of
these conditions, it may not be an emergency, but if you
ignore them, it may become an emergency.

134 Swelling of the Eye (Glaucoma)

This condition is rare in cats.

Causes
Failure of the fluid in the eye to circulate properly, resulting
in a rise in pressure inside the eye.

Symptoms
The eyeball increases in size and protrudes from the eye
socket. There is usually associated conjunctivitis and, in later
stages, corneal opacity (a milkiness of the eye).

Treatment
Glaucoma, like all eye conditions, must be treated only by a
professional. A vet will administer drugs to improve the
circulation of fluid. The only thing the cat owner can do is to
get the cat to a vet.

135 Tablets and Pills: Techniques of Administration

Concealment
If the cat is not being starved, conceal the pill or tablet in a

tasty titbit such as meat, cheese, or tuna fish.

Cats, however, are notorious for finding even the most cunningly concealed pill, and if this happens, be prepared to administer the pill directly.

Direct technique
(i)   Ideally, you should have an assistant. The assistant holds the cat, one hand on the scruff, the other arm wrapped round the cat's back legs.
(ii)   Place your left hand on top of the animal's head, with your thumb and index finger placed behind the canine teeth.
(iii)   Pull the cat's head backwards.
(iv)   The tablet is in your right hand. Use this hand to open the cat's mouth by holding the lower jaw behind the lower canine teeth.
(v)   Place the tablet at the back of the cat's throat.
(vi)   Hold the cat's jaw shut, until the animal licks its nose. When this happens, the cat has swallowed the tablet.

Unruly cats
(i)   Unruly cats should be first wrapped in a blanket or towel, with just the head showing.
(ii)   Slip a loop of bandage behind the lower canine teeth in order to pull the lower jaw down. The upper jaw is held by hand behind the upper canine teeth, as described above.
(iii)   An assistant administers the tablet by placing it at the back of the cat's throat.
(iv)   Alternatively, a tablet may be crushed between two tablespoons and the powder thrown to the back of the throat. This method is recommended only in especially difficult cases, since it may cause increased salivation, which works against the pill going down, and in fact may bring it up again.

---

136   Taking Samples of Faeces and Urine

Technique
To assist the vet in diagnosing certain illnesses, a specimen of the cat's faeces or urine will be needed.

Since cats do not always 'perform' at the most convenient time and place, this may require some persistence on the owner's part.

To collect urine from a cat, put a few spoonfuls of sand or

(i)

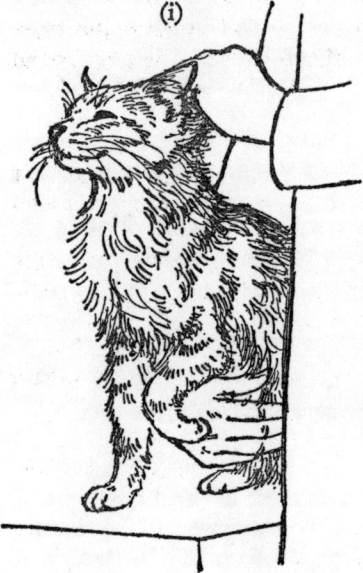

(ii) *and* (iii)

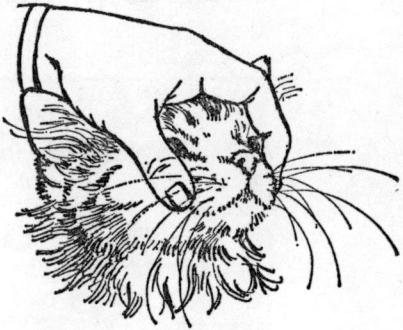

(iv)

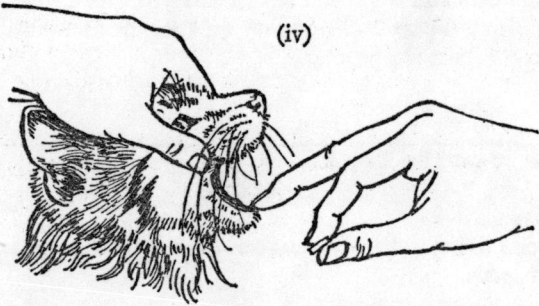

(v)

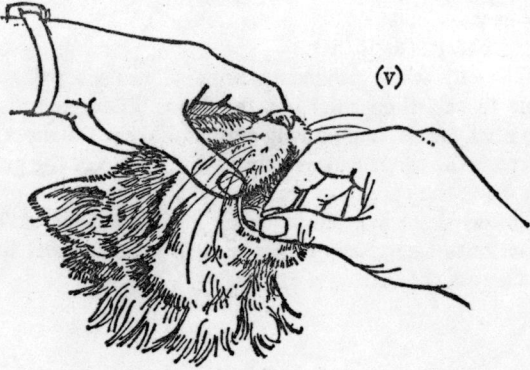

kitty litter in a cat tray, and then prop up one end of the tray so that the urine goes to that end. Be careful not to put in so much sand that it absorbs all the urine.

If your cat normally goes outdoors, keep it indoors until you have collected the sample.

Collect the urine or faeces immediately and put in a tin or bottle, clearly labelled with the cat's name, the owner's name, and the date.

Fortunately, one does not need a great deal of urine for laboratory analysis. A few drops will be sufficient.

---

137 Tar on the Feet

An occasional nuisance for owners of adventurous cats.

Treatment
(i) Bathe the cat's feet with a mixture of equal quantities of warm salt water and olive oil. Soak cotton wool in the mixture and gently rub the tar off the cat's feet. See **Restraint,** if necessary.
(ii) Whatever tar does not wash off during the foot bath should come off when you dry the cat's feet with a rag.
(iii) If all the tar does not come off after the first washing and drying, repeat the process.

---

138 Tartar on the Teeth

Causes
All cats living in hard water areas eventually develop tartar on their teeth.

Symptoms
1 Bad breath (halitosis).
2 The cat, while obviously hungry, refuses to eat; or it begins to eat, then spits out the food. There is usually excessive salivation, and pawing and rubbing at the mouth. This is because the tartar causes pain at the margin of the gums and teeth when the cat chews its food.
3 Should these symptoms occur, examine your cat's teeth. Tartar looks like crusts of kettle fur, which spread from the gums across the teeth.

Treatment
(i)   In hard water areas, give the cat boiled or distilled water to drink.
(ii)   With docile cats, during the early stages, tartar can be rubbed off with smoker's tooth powder. Remember, tartar accumulates on the back teeth as well as the front.
(iii)   In particularly stubborn cases, professional scaling by a vet may be necessary.

Prevention
Prevention of tartar accumulation can be accomplished by regular (about once a month) cleaning of the cat's teeth with either ordinary toothpaste on cotton wool, or by a little smoker's tooth powder on moist cotton wool.

Technique for cleaning teeth
Wrap the cat in a towel with only its head protruding. Then, with the cat tucked under your arm, lift the cat's lips and gently swab the moist cotton wool over the teeth. It may sound impossible, but in fact most cats do not mind having their teeth cleaned. After the first few times, they accept it as part of their regular grooming, and in some instances, they even co-operate.
  If cotton wool is difficult to manage, use a child's tooth-brush, which affords a bit more leverage.

---

139   Teething Stages in Kittens

Like humans, cats have two sets of teeth. The temporary teeth (or baby teeth) appear about three weeks after birth. These are replaced by the permanent teeth, which appear from five months onwards. As the permanent teeth push through the gums, they displace the temporary teeth which are either spat out or swallowed. By the sixth or seventh month, all the permanent teeth are in.
  Cats have twenty-six temporary teeth and thirty permanent teeth.

Care of teeth
(i)   Cats should have regular dental check-ups, by a vet, to prevent gingivitis, periodontitis, halitosis and eventual tooth loss.
(ii)   The wise owner will clean the cat's teeth regularly from

an early age with toothpaste or a little smoker's tooth powder on cotton wool.

There may be some problems in cleaning a cat's teeth; however, if the owner accustoms the cat to teeth cleaning while it is still very young, the habit will persist when the cat is grown.

140 Temperature Taking

Most infectious and contagious diseases in the early stages cause the body temperature to rise. The rise in body temperature is often, but not always, accompanied by lethargy and loss of appetite. Identification of temperature and its severity provides the cat owner with a guide as to whether a vet should be consulted.

Contrary to uninformed opinion, taking a cat's temperature is not at all difficult. The technique is very simple.

Type of thermometer
Any stubby, bulbed, clinical thermometer may be used. Such thermometers are available from all chemists.

Technique
A cat's temperature must always be taken by rectum. (If you put a thermometer in the cat's mouth, it will probably try to eat it.)

(i) Have someone hold the cat while you take its temperature (see **Restraint**). A well-trained pet should allow its owner to take its temperature without making too much of a fuss.

(ii) Hold the thermometer by the end opposite the bulb, between your index finger and thumb, and then shake it with a sharp jerky movement until the mercury is down to 95°F (35°C). (When you first do this, it is best to do it over a thick rug or bed, so that if you do drop the thermometer it will not break.)

(iii) Dip the bulb of the thermometer in vaseline, cold cream or baby oil.

(iv) Approach the cat from the rear, and gently slide 1 in (2·5 cm) of the thermometer through the anal sphincter, using a gentle rotary action. Be prepared to stop the cat from trying to sit down.

Cats are very conscious of their anal sphincters, and unless great care is taken, the animal may react violently and **you** may break the thermometer. So work it in gently.

Should the thermometer break, take the cat to a vet, if possible; if a vet is not available, administer liquid paraffin (*not kerosene*): 1 tablespoon (25 ml) orally, three times a day, until the thermometer is expelled with faeces.

(v) Push the thermometer in with a light touch, letting it find its own direction.

(vi) Once the thermometer is in place, support the protruding end very lightly and wait one full minute.

(vii) Then withdraw the thermometer, wipe it clean with cotton wool or kleenex and read the temperature.

Reading a thermometer

(i) All clinical thermometers are marked with large marks for each degree, and small marks for each fifth of a degree.

(ii) After withdrawing the thermometer from your cat, hold it up to the light and, still holding it by the end opposite the bulb, roll it between your fingers until you see the band of mercury.

(iii) Calculate the degree of temperature.

Normal body temperature
The normal body temperature of a cat is 101°F (38°C). Temperatures of 102.5°F (39°C) and higher are significant and good reason to consult a vet.

When calculating temperature, remember that an excited or frightened animal has a higher body temperature than a relaxed animal, so subtract a degree or two if this is the case.

When you have finished using the thermometer, wash it in cold water. Then sterilize it by dipping it in alcohol.

---

141 Ticks

Country animals quite often come into contact with the common sheep tick. Usually, ticks are first noticed when you are grooming your cat – another good reason for frequent grooming.

Description
The tick is a blood-sucking parasite with a shiny spherical body, varying in size from $\frac{1}{4}$ to $\frac{1}{2}$ in ($\frac{1}{2}$ to 1 cm) in diameter. The tick is creamy grey in colour. It looks something like a soya bean with tiny legs at one end.

Treatment
Do not try to pull the tick out. Ticks have powerful sucking jaws which are imbedded in the cat's skin. If you try to pull the tick out, its head will break off, leaving the mouth of the tick under the skin, and a sinus may eventually develop (a sinus is a small puncture wound which does not heal). The trick is to get the tick to remove its mouth *before* you pull it off your cat. There are three techniques for accomplishing this:

(i)   Pour a little ether or lighter fuel on to a pad of cotton wool, and place the pad over the tick for half a minute. Then pull the tick out.

(ii)   Smear each individual tick with vaseline and then remove it with tweezers.

(iii)   Hold the lighted end of a cigarette very close to the tick, without actually touching it or the cat. The heat will make the tick withdraw its head and it may then be removed.

If the head of the tick does break off
(i)   Clean the skin around the area with Cetavlon or soap and water.

(ii)   Using a boiled (sterile) needle, remove the head of the tick from under the cat's skin exactly as you would remove a splinter from your own finger.

(iii)   Dress the wound with a *poultice*.

In areas where ticks are common
In tick-infested areas, the cat can be kept free of ticks by bathing once a month in a ·0012 solution of benzene hexachloride (available from chemists). Be sure to wash all the solution off the cat's fur after bathing, since benzene hexachloride can be poisonous to cats. See **Restraint.**

---

142   Tonsillitis, Choking, Foreign Bodies in the Throat

These three conditions produce very similar symptoms.

General symptoms
1   The cat will cough, lick its lips, appear distressed and may cry out in pain. It will refuse food and may appear apathetic or sleepy.

2   Bones stuck between the larynx and the stomach cause no loss of appetite, but when the cat eats, it vomits. Also, there is

excessive dribbling and the cat will be profoundly depressed.
There is no home treatment for bones lodged in this area.
Professional assistance is necessary.

Treatment (foreign body in the throat or mouth)
(i)   First, open the cat's mouth and, with an electric torch,
look down its throat. See **Opening a Cat's Mouth.**
(ii)   If there is a foreign body, such as a bone, stuck in the
throat, use your fingers, or if it is too far down to reach, use a
pair of pliers to pull it out.

Symptoms of tonsillitis
1   The cat will appear to be choking.
2   When you open the cat's mouth, the tonsils, which are at
the back of the throat, will look like two swollen strawberry-
coloured lumps.
3   The cat will be very depressed.
4   The cat will have a high fever: temperature over 103°F
(39°C). See **Temperature Taking.**

Treatment of tonsillitis
(i)   Calm the cat with petting and soothing words. Then
administer one half of a Paracetamol tablet, once only. See
Tablets and Pills: Techniques of Administration.
(ii)   Give no food or water, except for some cracked ice, until
a vet has examined the cat. Cats with sore throats have a
tendency to vomit anything they swallow. If the cat is allowed
to fill its stomach with a quantity of water, it will retch and
further irritate its already irritated throat. This will make the
cat even thirstier, and will begin the dangerous Drink-Vomit
Cycle (see Index).
(iii)   Put the ice into a perforated bowl (a soap dish with
holes punched in it is ideal), so that the cat can moisten its
mouth by licking the ice, but cannot drink.

---

143   Tourniquets

The purpose of a tourniquet is to cut off the flow of blood
pumping from the heart out through a severed artery or vein.

In an emergency, a tourniquet can be improvised from
many things: a necktie, a belt, a strip of material, a shoe-lace,
even a strip of plaited grass will serve.

If the cat is bleeding badly, try to staunch the bleeding so that you can observe the way the blood is flowing: this indicates whether the cat is bleeding from an artery or a vein.

Arterial wounds
If the blood comes out in a pumping fashion, in time with the heartbeat, and is bright red, then it is from an artery and the bleeding must be stopped quickly or the cat will die.

For arterial wounds (on the limbs) make a tourniquet by wrapping the bandage or belt round the limb, above the injury. Then insert a pencil or screwdriver into the bandage. Twist the tourniquet until the bleeding stops.

Venous wounds
Blood flowing from a vein flows regularly, rather than being pumped out. The colour is dark red.

For venous wounds, apply the tourniquet below the wound and twist it until the bleeding stops.

General notes
Keep the tourniquet tight for not more than one minute. Then loosen it slightly.

Every ten minutes, loosen the tourniquet completely, to see whether the bleeding has stopped and to allow the blood to reach the rest of the leg and prevent tissue damage.

---

144 Trembling, Shivering

Causes
Cats shiver when they are:
1 frightened.
2 cold.
3 running a high fever.
4 over-excited.

Shivering or trembling that goes on for longer than half an hour is a sign that something is seriously amiss.

Examine the cat for fever.

Frightened cats pant as well as shiver.

---

145 Tumours

Tumours or cancers can affect any organ, system or part of the body at any age.

(i) Tourniquet for an arterial wound

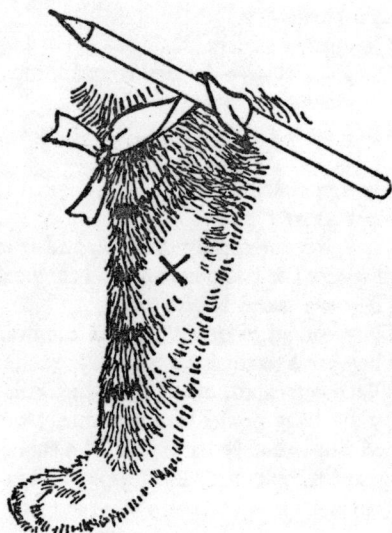

(ii) Tourniquet for a venous wound

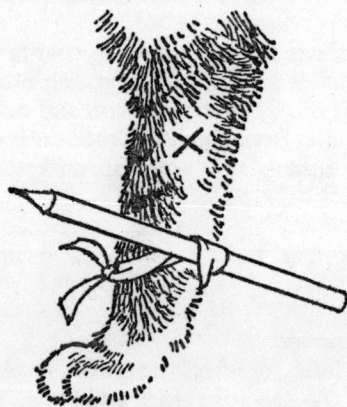

These tumours are divided into two groups, benign and malignant.

Benign tumours
1 They grow slowly.
2 They are clearly-defined round lumps.
3 They are cool to the touch.
4 They do not spread to other sites.

Malignant tumours
1 They grow rapidly.
2 They are not clearly defined, and it is sometimes difficult to tell where the tumour ends and the healthy tissue begins.
3 They are warm to the touch.
4 They spread to other parts of the body.
5 They tend to ulcerate.
6 If left untreated, eventually they kill.

Any swelling could be a tumour. Swellings should be examined immediately by a vet. The sooner the better. Even ·a malignant tumour may be stopped if it is caught early.

---

146   Unconsciousness

When you find a cat unconscious, unless the cause is *immediately apparent*, such as a great gaping wound, do not waste time looking for the cause. *The only exception to this is when the animal has been in contact with an electric wire* (see **Electric Shock**).

Just because the cat does not appear to be breathing, do not assume that it is dead, unless certain other factors are valid: the pupils dilate, the body is stiff and cold, there is no heartbeat or pulse. Even if you think the cat is dead and you cannot detect breathing, give artificial respiration for at least thirty minutes.

The reasons why cats lose consciousness may be divided into two very general categories: primary and secondary causes.

Primary causes
The cat loses consciousness as the result of a lesion (break) affecting the nervous system and brain. This occurs after car accidents or similar injuries, fits, strokes and narcosis produced by poisoning.

Secondary causes
The cat loses consciousness as the result of causes affecting other areas of the body. These include diabetic coma, uraemic coma (poison from the kidneys), calcium deficiency, shock, electric shock, drowning and heart attack.

Fainting causes
Cats faint if the blood supply to the brain is reduced or when it is deficient in oxygen. This occurs with cats which are in a state of shock, or whose hearts are not functioning properly.

Treatment
Cats which have fainted will recover spontaneously.
Make sure the animal's tongue is out and that nothing is blocking the windpipe. Most cats recover from faints in three or four minutes.

147 Urethral Obstructions; Bladder Stones (Cystic Calculi)

The urethra is the tube running from the bladder, through which urine is passed. This tube becomes irritated on occasion or, in severe cases, blocked. This condition is more prevalent in males.

Cause
Depending upon the seriousness of the symptoms, this condition could be caused by anything from a mild cystitis infection to bladder stones to complete blockage of the urethra. Blockage of the urethra is serious and must be treated immediately.

Symptoms
1 Inability to pass urine.
2 Squatting in litter box, as though constipated.
3 Distended abdomen.
4 Profound depression.

Treatment
There is no home treatment for this condition.

EMERGENCY
If your cat displays these symptoms, this is an emergency. You

*must have professional help immediately. Do not attempt to prod
the distended abdomen, or the bladder may rupture. If this
happens, the cat will die.*

148 Vaccination

Definition
A vaccine is an injection of substances (either living or dead
viruses) which provide immunity to certain virus or bacterial
diseases.

Natural immunity
Kittens receive antibodies from the first mother's milk, which
is called colostrum. This provides a natural immunity, which
lasts for eight to ten weeks and then diminishes.

In order not to interfere with this natural immunity, kittens
are usually not vaccinated until they are eight weeks old.

Orphan kittens
Orphan kittens which are being fed on supplement and have
not received colostrum, should be vaccinated at eight weeks
and again at twelve weeks of age to insure a high immunity.

Cat vaccines
Cats should be vaccinated to prevent infections of feline
enteritis, at twelve weeks of age.

149 Vomiting, Causes of

1 Infectious disease, e.g. feline enteritis.
2 Acute abdomen, e.g. peritonitis, intestinal obstruction.
3 Indigestion, e.g. overeating.
4 Metabolic disorders, e.g. nephritis.
5 Drugs, e.g. digitalis.
6 Nervous problems, e.g. motion sickness, fear.
7 Pharyngeal irritation, e.g. tonsillitis.
8 Poisoning.
9 Parasites.
10 Hernias.
11 Tumours.
12 Inflammation of the gullet.

150   Warts

Description
Small, pinkish, rounded lumps on the cat's skin.

Cause
The cause is not definitely known. Warts may be caused by a virus, or they may come from kissing frogs. In any case, they are not serious; and since they will not trouble your cat, do not let them trouble you.

Treatment
A wart has a definite neck and may be removed by the cat owner. Tie the wart off with a piece of cotton. In two or three days, the wart will drop off.
   Otherwise, warts are easily removed by a vet.

151   Weaning

Weaning is the process of taking a kitten off its mother's milk and putting it on to a diet of more adult foods.
   Kittens begin showing an interest in solid foods at three or four weeks old. This interest, however, does not mean that they are quite ready to be weaned. But their interest should be encouraged by offering them small amounts of finely chopped meat, boned fish or chicken and bowls of milk three or four times a day.
   When the kittens are five to six weeks old, they are ready to be weaned. At this time the mother begins to vomit her food (soft, partially digested) for her youngsters to eat.
   At about eight weeks of age, recently weaned kittens should be fed four meals a day (see **Diet**).

152   Weight

Increase in weight
A great increase in weight over a three to four week period is abnormal and suggests the possibility of one of the following:
1   Abdominal tumours.
2   General tumours.
3   Fluid in the abdomen (dropsy): certain serious diseases will cause the production of large amounts of fluid in the abdomen.

4 Compulsive eating, which may be the result of simple greed or brain damage.
5 Pregnancy.
6 Desexed cats tend to put on weight.
7 Thyroid deficiency.

Treatment
A definite diagnosis and treatment must be given by a vet. The above list is only a guide to the possible causes of a sudden increase in weight.

Loss of weight
A sudden loss of weight may be caused by:
1 Reduced intake of food.
2 Persistent vomiting.
3 Reduced absorption of food.
4 Tumours.
5 Chronic metabolic disease.

Treatment
The above list is a general guide to the possible causes of a sudden weight loss. If any of them are suspected, look them up in the Index and see if the symptoms described match those exhibited by your cat.

If you can identify the cause, although you will not be able to cure it, you may be able to treat the secondary symptoms as they arise. In any event, if there is continuing drastic weight loss, do not wait until the cat is down to fur and bones before you get professional assistance.

153 Worms

Worms are one of several types of parasite which may try to use your cat as host.

Unpleasant as they are, worms rarely cause serious problems, except in kittens. During the first eight months of the cat's life, the owner should be alert to the possibility of worms.

Causes
The worms are picked up from other animals and from the faeces of affected animals.

Symptoms

Worms in young cats produce a variety of symptoms. These may be seen separately or in association with each other.

1 Vomiting of worms.
2 Coughing.
3 Worms in the faeces.
4 A pot belly.
5 Halitosis.
6 Failure to grow correctly.

Adult symptoms

With adult cats, the presence of worms is rarely detected until the worms are either coughed up or appear in the faeces.

WARNING

While most types of worms are not particularly dangerous to the cat itself, the round worm can be transmitted to humans and may cause blindness. This is one good reason why children should not be encouraged to let stray kittens lick their faces, and a good reason to insist that they wash their hands before eating, and after playing with any animal, including their own.

Obviously, the differential diagnosis of worm infestations cannot be made by the cat owner. Therefore, it is advisable to treat all animals with suspected worm conditions with hygienic precautions.

Treatment

For worms other than tapeworm, administer piperazine tablets (available from chemists): 500 mg per 10 lb (5 kg) body weight. Repeat in one week.

Tapeworms

Symptoms

1 Tapeworms rarely cause any severe or dramatic symptoms, apart from a change in the texture and colour of the cat's coat. The coat will become dry, dull and out of condition.
2 There may be some non-specific illness, and diarrhoea. By 'non-specific' illness we mean that the cat may be off form: nothing you can put your finger on, just not well.
3 The observant owner will notice segments of tapeworms in the faeces, and stuck to the fur around the anus.

Description
The cat owner will have no difficulty in distinguishing the
tapeworms; indeed, it would be difficult not to distinguish
them.

When freshly passed, these segments are about $\frac{1}{4}$ in ($\frac{1}{2}$ cm)
long, moist and quite active. They dry rapidly and
shrivel up. When dry, they resemble small brownish grains of
rice. These dried-up tapeworms are often found in the cats
bedding.

Treatment
Fortunately, treatment is simple and usually effective. There
are a number of excellent commercial tapeworm preparations
available e.g. Dichlorophen. Administer 500 mg per 6 lb (3 kg)
body weight after a meal. Then wait seven days and repeat the
dose.

Since tapeworms are carried by fleas, get rid of the fleas as
well as the tapeworms. See **Fleas.**

---

154   Wounds

A wound is a break or 'lesion' of the body surfaces. When the
wound occurs, the cat bleeds. If the wound is superficial and
the bleeding slight, in the normal course of events the blood
will clot and the bleeding will stop. But if the cat is losing a lot
of blood, first aid must be administered.

Treatment
The first priority is to stop the bleeding, irrespective of
whether or not it is arterial or venous.

(i)   If the animal is bleeding very badly, do not waste time:
jam a wad of rags, tissues or a towel over the wound, press
hard and hold the wad of material there until the bleeding
stops. If nothing else is available, use your hand or fingers
pressed directly on to the wound to stop the bleeding.

(ii)   Once you have staunched the wound, try to determine
whether it is arterial or venous. If the blood is bright red and
spurting, it comes from a severed artery. If the blood is a
deeper red and oozing, it comes from a vein.

(iii)   For arterial wounds, apply a tourniquet between the
wound and the heart.

(iv)   For venous wounds, the tourniquet is applied on the side
of the wound farthest from the heart.

(v)   If the wound is on the trunk, or on the neck, where a tourniquet cannot be used, you will have to keep pressing the wad of material or your hand over the wound until the bleed-stops. When you do remove the pressure, be careful not to tear away the protective clotting and start the bleeding again.

(vi)   Once the bleeding has been controlled, the next step depends on the severity of the injury and whether or not the cat is in a state of shock. If not, proceed to treat the wound.

Dressing the wound

(i)   Clip the hair around the wound with blunt-ended scissors.

(ii)   Wash the wound with soap (any good-quality hand soap) and cooled boiled water. If you have an antiseptic, such as Cetavlon or Dettol, use it. Otherwise, just soap and water will do. Be sure to wash away any dirt, oil or grease from the centre of the wound.

(iii)   After drying, apply a simple dressing to keep out infection. A pad of cotton wool secured with elastoplast will do the job. Change the dressing once a day, See **Bandaging.**

(iv)   For severe wounds, after cleaning and dressing, contact a vet.

Classification of wounds

The most efficacious treatment for a wound can be deduced from observing the type of wound it is.

Clean, incised wounds

These bleed freely and a pressure bandage or tourniquet may be applied.

Lacerated wounds

These are jagged irregular wounds, which bleed minimally and require ordinary bandaging.

Puncture wounds

These are usually caused by bites and are almost always infected. See **Abscesses.**

Contused wounds

These may be any of the above types of wounds which are accompanied by surrounding bruises. In addition to washing and disinfecting the wound, hot compresses should be applied. See **Compresses, Cold and Hot.**

Chest wounds

Treatment

Place a moistened pad or wad of material directly over the wound.

If there are any plastic bags or sheets of polythene available, place these over the pad and hold them in place with elastoplast or ordinary sticky-tape to obtain an airtight shield over the wound.

In an emergency, do not waste time looking for a pad or wad of material. Use your hand or fingers to stop the bleeding. Put your hand or fingers directly on to the bleeding wound, and press. This should stop the bleeding until you can get a proper dressing on to the wound.

Do not remove the dressing.

If a wound continues to bleed through a dressing, apply another pad and bandage it tighter; or apply more pressure by hand over the wound. Do not remove the first dressings; this will only disturb the blood clot which is forming over the wound, and make the bleeding worse.

Transporting a cat with a chest wound

(i)   Move a wounded cat only when you have to.

(ii)   If you can hear the air sucking in and out of the wound, then carry the cat on its breastbone. If not, carry the animal with the wound uppermost.